Florence Ditlow is an amazing woman with an incredible story to tell. *Long in the Tooth* will both inspire and delight the reader. This is a story of a very courageous woman coping with a strange and mysterious disease. Every step along the way she meets each difficulty with a sense of joy, whimsy and playfulness. You will laugh and you will cry. Even though she faces a life threatening illness, Florence greets each new day with hope, determination and a strong will to live. Her story is proof that "A merry heart does good like a medicine". I am certain that both Norman Cousins and Patch Adams would choose Florence as their "poster girl" for the healing power of humor and laughter.

Patty Wooten RN
Author of *Compassionate Laughter—Jest for Your Health*.
Lifetime Achievement Award winner for her pioneering work in therapeutic humor

Long in the Tooth is an inspiring autobiography of a courageous nurse diagnosed with ALS. She uses her medical knowledge and embarks on a six-year journey toward healing. She frankly discusses the exploration of her spirituality and the power of love. This is a story about a woman who comes to understand the use of humor, alternative medicine, and insight as means to banish pain and to gain control over her life. The author discovers the power of forgiveness as she opens herself to the past, and the promise of a loving marriage as she frees herself from her fear of the future. The author writes about the psychological effects of chronic illness – the discomfort, the depression, and the depletion of energy. Ms. Ditlow discusses therapeutic approaches that may be helpful to others dealing with neurological illnesses. I am eagerly awaiting her next book.

Ellen M. Carter, MSW, LCSW

Long in the Tooth

Long in the Tooth

▼

Surviving Chronic Illness with a Sense of Humor

Florence Ditlow

Writers Advantage
New York Lincoln Shanghai

Long in the Tooth
Surviving Chronic Illness with a Sense of Humor

All Rights Reserved © 2002 by Florence Ditlow

No part of this book may be reproduced or transmitted in any form or by any means, graphic, electronic, or mechanical, including photocopying, recording, taping, or by any information storage retrieval system, without the written permission of the publisher.

Writers Advantage
an imprint of iUniverse, Inc.

For information address:
iUniverse
2021 Pine Lake Road, Suite 100
Lincoln, NE 68512
www.iuniverse.com

Consult your healthcare practitioner before attempting the practices outlined here.

ISBN: 0-595-24771-7

Printed in the United States of America

For Genady, who taught me that love wins the game.

Preface

▼

Long in the Tooth, is a true account of my response to the dangers inherent in the heavy metals used in dentistry. People who are sensitive to mercury, tin, copper, and other metals used in dental amalgams, may be subject to a host of autoimmune diseases. This book is about how I survived an exposure to these toxic metals. I intend that my effort to shed light on the problem will spare others this unnecessary experience. The *prescription* I designed in response to my illness is outlined here: not as a formula for others, but as an example. It is one person's choice from the dozens of alternative therapies available.

I wrote about this topic from the point of view of the person coping with the illness. My career of thirty years as a registered nurse did not prepare me for the problems that I faced in detoxifying my system.

My story is about saying yes to a happy and healthy future. It is designed to serve the multitude of people facing any chronic illness, who want the best body they are able to have. I also know that humor is a saving grace; that no matter how dark the path of life gets, humor is infinitely available.

Acknowledgements

▼

In addition to those mentioned in *Long in the Tooth*, I would like to express my gratitude to the following helpful people, and to the countless strangers who have opened countless doors. My patients' names have been changed for the purpose of confidentiality:

Bikram Yoga, Bruce Baar, Rev. Jeannie Brannon, Christopheray, Bob Cicione, C.S.W., Louise Ditlow, Dr. Allan Douglas, Mike Feder, Ella Filkovsky, Leonid Filkovsky, Ph.D., Judy Gire, Rev. Greg Hagin, Norma Keider Ph.D., Donna Laino-Curran, R.N., Dr. Jay Lombard, Ruth Kaciak, New York City Transit Paratransit, Joan McLaughlin, Trudy Meehan, Yvonne Naum, Ph.D., New Jersey Transit, Myriam Orozco, Barbara Pittman, R.N., Adrian Ramm, Susan Sagui L.M.T., Dr. Vimal Sharda, Terry Spano, Anelle Stanislas, Barry Strutt, Simon Taffler, Terry Tober, Alfonso Valdiva, Andrea Versenyi, C.S.W., Steven Weiss, D.O., Stephan Wischerth, and Joyce Woullard, L.P.N.

Leslie Li was especially important in the creation of "Long in the Tooth". Her seminar for writers convinced me to write this book.

Photography by Ian Couch

Contents

▼

Preface	ix
Long in the Tooth: Surviving Chronic Illness with a Sense of Humor	1
1994	3
The Wedding	11
Humor Therapy	16
Laughing with Patients	20
1995: An End and a Beginning	43
1995 Continued	56
1996	65
Panchakarma	73
Fancy Channeling	78
Energy	85
Dental Metals: The Missing Link	93
1997	97
The Subway Healings	107
1998	113
Bodywork and Supportive Therapies	119
1999	124
Long distance transmissions	128
2000	131
2002	133
Humoring the Patient When the Patient is Me	135
References	141

Word Index 145
Author's Biography 151

Long in the Tooth: Surviving Chronic Illness with a Sense of Humor

▼

"The world is so overflowing with absurdity that it is difficult for the humorist to compete."

Malcolm Muggeridge

The Q train was on time and I was a minute late. I heard it coming through the subway tunnel to the Roosevelt Island, New York, stop, as I walked down the moving escalator. Shifting into a run, I cleared the moving stair, heard the train stop, and flying down the last short stairwell, I heard a man racing behind me as we jumped through the closing doors. The race for the train felt so good. I wasn't even out of breath.

"Thanks for running," he puffed. "I couldn't hear the train coming…didn't want to miss it."

I smiled. That was in 1993, the last time I ran for the train.

I mentally replayed my weekend as the 3:05 train pulled out, taking me to work. My family had completed a two-day hike in the White Mountains— now that was exhilarating. The first day we trekked at least ten miles, over sparkling streams and jagged granite, while listening to Genady's kids, Yana, and Eyal, argue about who was the better hiker.

"Real hikers have walking sticks."

"Real hikers don't run out of water."

"Real hikers know how to keep bears away."

"Shut up…real hikers don't have to explain why they're real."

The vista from our destination that day was a clear assortment of green valleys, mixed with granite-laced mountains, nothing in that view was man made. We had just about half a mile to go. I felt more tired, with each passing pine tree, and hungrier with each passing boulder. I would welcome the warmth of the cloud-hidden Appalachian Mountain Club cabin, where we had reserved bunks. Sitting at a weather beaten picnic table, shedding my backpack, suddenly, my left leg began to shake involuntarily. It only jerked spasmodically for half a minute, but this neuromuscular event foreshadowed upcoming adventures that would change everything.

1994

▼

Dream…

I meet a large group of nurses, who say that they run a Summer Camp. Looking around, I see that the kids in this camp number a quiet, two.

"Wow!" I remarked. "You're not really working."

"Nooooo," said one in a whisper.

"We're resting. Recovering. Vegging out," said the other, in a calm voice that could hypnotize. "And I'm not joking."

I interpreted the dream as a sign to think about resigning my nursing position; working as a staff R.N., in a city hospital. In my waking hours, I had been making arrangements for our wedding.

I had had a rather long prenuptial engagement with the man who is my best friend, Genady. We were waiting for his parents to be able to attend the wedding. They were moving to this country from the Middle East. Late in 1993, while setting our marital machine in motion, I decided to check out some physical symptoms, which appeared to have a neurological origin.

First, I had tests, which would diagnose my recent swallowing difficulties. The pharyngeal symptoms included difficulty swallowing and speaking. I had been coping with excessive amounts of saliva, and gum disease, which had been present since 1991.

I was more concerned about finding the cause of a sudden lack of coordination, and imbalance. I had fallen three times, in the past six months. Were these accidents? My ear, nose and throat physician referred me to a neurologist, a slight man, who never altered his mask of concern.

He performed many tests, and to my questions about possible diagnoses, he replied, "I'll reserve judgment until I see all the test results."

The magnetic resonance imaging was done to see a map of the brain and to provide evidence that there was not a tumor hiding behind the symptoms. Electromyograms, or EMGs, are tests of muscular contraction, important in diagnosis of neurological diseases.

The EMG is a great thing, probably invented by a sadist. It involves the insertion of needles into various muscles. These wonderful needles are connected to a machine, which measures electrical activity.

After meeting with the neurologist, blood tests were done, and while I waited in the doctor's lab, I pulled a large medical book off the shelf, turning to the section on neuron disease: Amyotropic Lateral Sclerosis. The text blurred as I read, "life expectancy two to five years."

At one point, (no pun intended) as the doctor inserted a needle into my neck, I got the idea to try acupuncture.

"You're probably acquainted with acupuncture," I said, wincing with pain.

"I don't know anything about it, and I don't want to know," he retorted.

I thought this seemed a hidebound, narrow-minded attitude. I began to wonder about him. Soon, I was in his fluorescent, cubical office, as he, in his words, was "giving" me the diagnosis, not unlike "giving me" an infection. His manner was abrupt. He said, "You have ALS, Amyotropic Lateral Sclerosis."

ALS is better known as Lou Gherig's disease. Later, I thought, there are few diseases with *disease* in the name. My world came to a screeching halt.

"You have ALS, and, as an R.N., you know what that implies."

Did it imply that I would be like others with neurological weaknesses: totally dependent on others for feeding, clothing and care?

Did this imply multiple doctor visits, followed by exponential suffering in a prison-like life, in a wheel chair? Did this imply that I would have to see this nincompoop again?

My mind drifted back to an ALS patient, a friend, who was a woman diagnosed at the age of seventy. Mildred had dropped her house key while attempting to turn it in the door lock of her house. After other subsequent muscular weaknesses, her respiratory muscles finally failed, and she was gone. The whole process from the day the key dropped until she died, took less than one year!

I couldn't think. I remembered the feeble Mildred, in her hospital bed, as the neurologist behind his steel desk droned on.

"You'd do well to enter a research program…you could get experimental medication as well as physical therapy."

"I'm sorry to have to give you this diagnosis. I did meet one patient who recovered," he said flatly, as he handed over a prescription for ankle braces, physical therapy, and a speech evaluation.

I leaned forward, emerging from my trance. "He recovered? How? Who was he?"

"One day he came to tell me at the clinic that all his symptoms disappeared."

"I'd love to talk to him!" I replied, grasping for hope.

"It's been so long and I don't remember his name."

I sighed, and thought, "I'll have your license taken away before you hurt another person! Why, this is 'emotional' malpractice." Exiting the office door, I silently screamed, "He hurt me! He didn't help!"

I walked from the west side of town, soon entering the sunny, south side of Central Park, and sat on a park bench, near a sheltering oak tree. I deeply breathed the smell of newly unfurled tree leaves. I was one of a few people there that spring day. The soothing songs of the robins as they bobbed near me were most welcome. I stared at the pool of clouds reflected in the water nearby. Within a few minutes, I actually witnessed a Blue Heron, as he landed in the water.

His landing in the tranquil pool brought me back from my own pool of negativity. I mentally waded back to the real world and saw that I was in a nature sanctuary.

So I sat on that park bench, in shock, wondering where to turn, when a man appeared, who looked quite familiar. He had been a regular attendee at the *Comic Relief*, humor group I belonged to, and led.

I had been meeting with homeless people to promote laughter as a therapeutic experience, volunteering my skills as a psychiatric nurse, and humor therapist for three years.

A homeless man, Burt Richterman, whom I had chanced to meet on a subway train, started the group. He named the group; *Comic Relief*, after the telethon for homeless people of the eighties, by the same name, hosted by Robin Williams, Whoopee Goldberg, and Billy Crystal.

Exercising our sense of humor is one of the best activities available to us as fellow humans. It's good effects seem to multiply when that humor is shared with a group of people.

In the sixties, writer, Norman Cousins, defined humor as therapy. He believed humor to be more than laughter. "Humor," he said, "contains hope, faith, determination, festivity, love, and the will to live." I went to *Comic Relief* in order to deliver a therapeutic group experience. Humor could be seen as a form of mind-body medicine. Our group has laughed at life's tragedies and laughed for the joy of surviving another day. We've laughed at videos, which evoked good memories planted by the comedians of yesteryear. We did role-playing for stressful encounters such as job interviews, videotaped it, and laughed. I urged them to develop an *eye* for humor, that is, to see the humor surrounding us. Such an exercise involved walking out to various businesses as secret agents, and searching for humor in their public relations. The homeless veterans have repeatedly shown me how humor has the power to lift the spirit, and they often did that without support of a paycheck, a home, or a family.

Al smiled through his rotten teeth, framed by a gray beard. Tipping his Yankee cap, he greeted me with a handshake, and took a seat on the bench. I was reeling after the encounter with the neurologist, whose diagnostic delivery rang over and over in my ear, like a skipping record. I must have looked like I had seen my own ghost. I felt fear, but I could not explain it to Al. The words were too large to process. They would have gotten stuck in my throat. I listened to Al's vagabond tales, and as he rambled on about his wasted life, unknowingly he comforted me. I found myself telling him about a favorite cartoon, by Kliban, captioned: "Wasted and useful lives." It shows two frames. In the first frame, there is a professional man, sweating at a desk, doing a nine-to-five job. The second frame shows a bearded drunk on an island, leaning against a palm tree, watching native dancing girls.

After an hour of listening to Al, I seemed to regain my sanity. We left the park to walk down Fifth Avenue. We both had appointments to keep. As I walked, I stepped into an altered state. Perhaps it was Al's eerily angelic connection, or perhaps it was my deranged endorphins. I was sensing life as a web of consciousness. I felt intense suffering, from the man sitting on the sidewalk in rags, to the baby, running, and then falling down in front of me. I felt hot, as a couple of elderly ladies, with heavy winter coats, crept along in front of the New York Public Library. I was one with each of my fellow human beings in their search for autonomy, because now, my own freedom, and independence were at stake.

Twenty blocks from Central Park, I bid farewell to Al, who was going in the opposite direction. The last time I saw him was when he entered the Fortieth Street subway station.

I wish I could have told him what an angel he was on that day. He had gently repaired what the neurologist had damaged in my spirit.

My appointment, a most important one, was at Lord and Taylor. I entered the department store with its festive green and white awning, and stood among a few old ladies who were clutching their shopping bags. Then I proceeded to think about death. Death. Nature's way of holding your calls indefinitely.

To grow old is to win, I thought, that's the name of the game. I didn't know it at the time, but I was about to begin releasing the fear that had been planted by the neurologist.

I started with the *Scarlett O'Hara*, stress reduction method. It has the same effect as whistling in the dark: "I can't think about this now, I'll go crazy if I do. I'll think about this tomorrow. For after all, tomorrow *is* another day." For authenticity, I thought in a southern accent.

Then these thoughts turned to the reason I had come to Lord and Taylor. It was to meet Genady, my future husband. I had an appointment to be fitted for my wedding dress! I could imagine myself speaking on the phone, to my mother, saying,

"Oh what a day! I started out at the doctor's office, being diagnosed with a life threatening disease, and then I bought my wedding dress."

These thoughts precipitated into hot, angry tears, when Genady came through the revolving door. He was smiling at the end of a tiring workday. I sniffed through the tale of the nincompoop, and his diagnosis.

While we stood holding each other in the jewelry section, I was grateful that no salespeople were around, to suspect that we were some pitiful couple, breaking our engagement at the diamond counter.

"Honey," he said in his deep voice, behind a look of concern, "You're going to be OK."

He took a tissue and wiped the puddle of tears off the jewelry counter glass, to reveal rows of diamond solitaires.

"You don't have to marry me," I said, now that I was breathing regularly again.

"Honey!" he admonished.

"People with ALS require lots of care," I argued, "and it's not fair to you."

I described Stephen Hawking to him, but he reminded me wisely that even bad problems have solutions. Genady must see all of life's problems as bugs in computer programs. Debugging is his specialty.

Finally, he reduced me to another round of tears, but these were tears of joy, accompanied by a shaky smile.

"Honey," he said, holding me, "however you are, I love you. I want to marry you."

I carefully decided not to take the neurologist's advice to enter an experimental research program. I had phoned, seeking information about the free study program offered by an ALS center. I was told matter-of-factly, that I would have physical therapy, an experimental drug called Riluzol, and muscular strength measurements. In 1994, Riluzol was credited with the extension of the lives of a group of ALS patients. The picture that was painted wasn't pretty, but perhaps I would have had the benefit of a neurologist who wasn't a nincompoop.

My past medical experience combined with intuition, weighed the effort involved, versus the benefits. I needed to be surrounded by a healing environment. After thirty years in nursing, I knew that there is never only one right way to improve your health. Many options existed—now I needed to choose the best one for myself.

Instead of the ALS research program, I located a woman neurologist, Dr. Chan, who was not associated with the neurologist who gave me the first opinion. She was Chinese, which was not an accident. I discovered her when an acquaintance, trained in acupuncture, urged me to try it. The acupuncturist shared an office with my new neurologist.

Dr. Chan was a fast moving, middle-aged woman, who wore eyeliner to emphasize her smiling eyes.

I eagerly awaited her thoughts about my situation, which were somewhat refreshing.

"I have to agree with your previous physician," she said, "because I'm sure you haven't got Multiple Sclerosis, Muscular Dystrophy, or a brain tumor. That leaves one choice: ALS. That said, you don't fit the typical ALS picture. You are doing too well!"

She put me on the same drug, Riluzol, used in the research center, and asked me to be part of a clinical trial. I walked out of her office feeling grateful for having found someone as kind and knowledgeable as she. I didn't care for the nincompoop, but he did set me in motion, although it was a rude awakening. I would proceed with acupuncture treatments, if only because the nincompoop didn't agree with its use.

My acupuncturist was born in Europe, unlike her Chinese counterparts in the acupuncture clinic. After I described my symptoms along with the two medical opinions, Eva Berend shook her head.

"Most of my time here is spent undoing the harm caused by Western doctors."

"I'm willing to work at getting well, but…but…there's so little help out there! I believed that doctors had learned how to empower patients but…I assumed too much," I sniffed.

"I believe there are things which can help," said Eva. "You will prove them wrong."

With that pleasant thought, she proceeded to insert hair-thin needles, painlessly, from head-to-toe. Acupuncture had no obvious effect on my balance, but I had an unexpected improvement in my appetite. I failed to notice that my appetite had all but disappeared. After Eva's treatment, I enjoyed eating meals again. I think acupuncture also helped me to loosen the knot of fear, which was associated with the initial diagnosis of ALS.

Acupuncture needles can stimulate the flow of blood and oxygen to the area of treatment, causing muscular relaxation. Cellular energy for healing is liberated, which the Chinese refer to as *chi*. The rebalancing effect of acupuncture, enhances immunity, and I was sure that I needed to build a strong immune system.

I had a short series of five treatments, before my acupuncturist moved out of town. I decided to try acupuncture, about six months later at a different office. I went for treatment every two weeks for a year, but stopped due to inclement weather.

During this phase of my illness, which called for self-sustaining strategies, I saw my chiropractor, Joe Adler, and explained my situation. He reminded me of the power of the human body, and that I should attempt to tune into it. Woven through his life-affirming words was a theme, which was slowly beginning to crystallize: *trust yourself*.

The Wedding

▼

This marriage be wine with halvah, honey dissolving in milk.
This marriage be the leaves and fruit of a date tree.
This marriage be women laughing together for days on end.
This marriage be a sign for us to study.
This marriage beauty.
This marriage a moon in a light blue sky.
This marriage this silence fully mixed with spirit.

    Rumi

Despite my health crisis and the attendant anxiety, I enjoyed the prelude to the wedding: setting the dates, conferring with the minister, and selecting the menu for the reception. Genady was thrilled at the prospect of the event, and wrote much of the ceremony, focusing upon friendship. We took books of poetry from our own shelf, and selected quotes from Rumi, and Gibran. These we would read to each other in the service. We would wed in Harrisburg, Pennsylvania, in July. The setting we chose for the post-nuptials was the Hershey Hotel, Hershey, PA, the self-acclaimed sweetest place on Earth, where the *Chocolate Kiss* is manufactured.

  We bought our gold rings from a friend, Durga Katz, whom I had met while learning to market the humor therapy skills. She specialized in one-of-a-kind pieces, sold in her apartment on the west side.

  "Do you have anything that looks important?" I asked her, casting a glance at my *love*, who was trying on a selection of plain gold bands.

After looking at several jeweled rings, we singled out a very imposing gold band, with one recessed solitaire. The ring had one border of square cutouts, resembling those atop a castle. In many cultures, geometric shapes symbolize life's passages. Various folklores of the world often use geometric shapes as symbols in storytelling. I thought of this as we bought the rings. Genady was enamored of the square, while I related more to the circle. A mathematician by training, he was adept at factoring things in, and tying things down. The ring, which contained both a square border and a square cut diamond, appealed to his sense of order. The ring combined his *squared* stability with my *circular* process.

I wanted to come full circle into wholeness. With Genady as my soul mate, I earnestly desired that life would follow a rhythmical cycle, one where we could predict future activities, unhindered by the limitations of ill health. I dared to be filled with hope.

Weddings are a great excuse to celebrate the joining of forces. Ours brought together relations and friends to the Unitarian church in Harrisburg, PA, that agreed to join a sometime Unitarian, with a man who describes himself as a non-religious Jew. The local rabbi had a problem joining two people of differing faiths. The Episcopal Church of my childhood refused to marry us, because I had strayed from the Anglican Church as an adult.

Why not break all the rules? After all, our choice of attire had been a joint venture, why not get dressed together? The dress I stepped into had cream-colored layers of silk, which floated over a mid-calf, pleated skirt. The spool-heeled shoes had long, pointy, fairy godmother toes, and I stepped to the mirror gingerly, to test my stability. Genady pulled on his white tux jacket, which complemented his olive skin.

"Is it OK?" Genady asked, raising an eyebrow at his tux.

I kissed him. "Yes. You are the best. Please go slowly out there. Jim will be taping this," I said, referring to my brother, "and I'd rather not be filmed while tripping."

"Don't worry, honey, if you fall down, I'll fall too, and we'll pretend it's a Unitarian mating ritual."

Rather than wear a veil, I chose a headband of multicolored rosebuds. He adjusted my crown as we proceeded to the church, where our thirty wilting guests had convened.

At the first piano strains of Pachebel's *Canon*, we walked hand-in-hand to the front of the church, and took our places in front of an altar, which was a brick wall. Candles added to the sweltering heat, in the silence broken only by a buzzing fan. The guests craned their necks, peering over their shoulders in anticipation of the minister, who finally entered.

When he finally appeared, we began reading from Gibran:

On Friendship

And a youth said, Speak to us of Friendship.
And he answered, saying:
Your friend is your needs answered.
He is your field which you sow with love
and reap with thanksgiving.
And he is your board and fireside.
For you come to him with your hunger,
and you seek him for peace.
...And let your best be for your friend.
If he must know the ebb of your tide,
let him know its flood also.
For what is your friend that you should
seek him with hours to kill?
Seek him always with hours to live.
For it is his to fill your need
but not your emptiness.
And in the sweetness of friendship let
there be laughter, and sharing of pleasures.

For in the dew of little things the heart
finds its morning and is refreshed.

Our guests participated, interjecting words of encouragement. If they only knew how much I needed to hear them, not so much for the validation of our well-established love and friendship, but for my very life.

"Inside this new love, die. Become the sky. Walk out like someone suddenly born into color."

Rumi

We were married in 1994, on the same day the comet, Shoemaker-Levy, collided with Jupiter. To us it seemed as though the entire universe rejoiced. We spent our honeymoon in Bermuda, in a musty, colonial mansion, which provided a pool, perfumed by the surrounding shocking pink hibiscus.

The breakfast portion of our bed and breakfast was an amusing adventure, that is, if you like breakfast. Each morning, a Philippine gentleman, unfailingly recited the same menu, in his singsong voice.

"Coffee, tea, juice…toast…and Rice Krispies!"

One by one, the guests who knew the menu by heart, would impatiently interrupt his breakfast song, saying, "Just coffee…please!"

Our colonial mansion was a bike ride from the ocean. Often, we rented bikes and cycled on Bermuda's dirt roads. I immediately discovered that my equilibrium would be sorely tested, when I crashed into a hedge on our dirt path. Luckily, the trails were lined with soft, brushy, tropical plants, which cushioned my inevitable impact with the ground.

"Well," I said, puffing, "if I go slowly enough, I can lean into these hedges and use them as a kind of net."

As we headed toward the beach, Genady followed closely and picked me out of the hedge after the initial spin and spill. My nerves performed better after that. Practice, and a formerly excellent kinesthetic sense, combined to make the rides possible. The scratches and bruises were worth it;

worth standing in pink sand, and morning ocean spray, and worth being able to absorb purple and orange sunsets.

"Snap. Crackle. Pop." On the third day, I began reciting the menu on the way to the dining room. Genady asked for jam. Surprisingly, it was on the menu, and that was a new experience.

After breakfast this sunny day, leaving Genady to pursue underwater sports, I headed for the beach, where I discovered a cave-like, black rock formation. A woman, whom I chanced to meet, informed me that the rocks, which lined the beach and jutted out of the ocean here and there, were black coral and good for us, in that they absorbed negativity. Left inside the cool safety of the rock, I communed with crabs, and a few beach flies, and painted my first, small, watercolor view of the ocean. Saltwater colors, I called them, as I mixed pigment with ocean water.

Here, ocean merged seamlessly with sky. This was a long abandoned art and it acted upon my neurological nightmare like a charm. Brushes washed, I turned to stare at the ocean, unlimited by personal responsibility or by work schedules.

That the humor in my soul emerged on our trip, was proved by the motorbike ride for two. I saw that it was raining, and donned a transparent, hooded plastic poncho. This hood needed something to attach it to my head, so I employed a very strange pair of black sunglasses, sliding them over my ears, thus keeping the plastic hood in place. Genady laughed uncontrollably at the black plastic lenses, which were asymmetrical, with one oval being vertical, and one horizontal. The rain added hilarity to the ride, my plastic tail flying behind us.

> The minute I heard my first love story
> I started looking for you, not knowing
> how blind that was.
> Lovers don't finally meet somewhere.
> They're in each other all along.
>
>   Rumi

Humor Therapy

▼

"Life is like photography; you need the negative to develop."

Swami Beyondananda

Are love and humor related? There is no doubt in my mind that they are. I was introduced to humor therapy in 1985, the same year the Challenger spacecraft exploded. Shortly afterward, I experienced another explosive event, when the nursing division at Knoxville's East Tennessee Baptist Hospital, was informed that any of us could be downsized, forced into part-time hours, or reassignment to different areas of the hospital. A five-minute meeting, a few months later with an associate nursing director, turned out to be the unceremonious finale to my sixteen years of service.

Seething with fury at having been dumped, I proceeded to search for work. It was within this dark, negative feeling state, that humor lightly tapped me on the shoulder. It came when I discovered a group of nurses who promoted the use of humor in the face of a wide array of stress. I certainly needed to laugh. I realized that holding onto the anger that stemmed from the loss of my work, income, and identity, was not harming anyone but me. I soon decided to laugh out the negative, and to do so regularly. For a five-dollar membership fee, I became one of the *Nurses for Laughter*. Along with the membership, I received a large button labeled in red letters: WARNING: Humor may be hazardous to your illness.

After a succession of temp jobs, in Knoxville, I accepted a full-time position in Boston, at the prestigious Massachusetts Eye and Ear

Infirmary, where I worked alongside a group of other stressed-out nurses. I decided to share my interest in humor with the nursing vice-president, and nurse-managers, who by the way, were filled with humor. I would go to different floors in a brief, weekly humor crusade. I would do it for a year, in the hope of building a laugh support group, a coterie of *believers*. I envisioned that we would find a way to bring humor to ourselves and to our patients.

I began my *humor rounds* by visiting different floors of the hospital, meeting with nurses at the shift change. There, I spent a few minutes doing something to break through the stress-shells we all wore. Sometimes I related jokes I had been told by our patients, and sometimes I played excerpts from comedy tapes, brought in clownish toys, or encouraged inane tests proving how good their humor was. Then there were the songs, such as the following, set to the tune of "Side by Side."

Oh we don't think infection is funny
even less those sores that are runny
But we are all quick
to prevent getting sick
Wash your hands!

Before leaving, I handed out laughter research, showing how the body and mind benefit from the release of stress hormones. It showed that blood pressure readings respond to laughing as they do to other aerobic exercise, though unlike the health club, laughter is free. The nurses read about catecholamines, the hormone build-up of stress, and how laughter could drive out this harmful residue. They saw in print the evidence that humor also has a *leveling effect*. In other words, that it places people on the same level, regardless of age, social status or race. My colleagues thought it was nice, but not nice enough to consider providing humor to patients. "We can use a laugh as much as anyone," they told me, "but we don't have any time or energy to devote to it."

I learned much that year: that humor was needed by nurses themselves, how to run group sessions, and I learned that I needed humor more than ever. Being single, with no prospects for companionship, I decided to go on *humor dates*. A humor date guarantees humor. It means treating oneself as well as possible, dressing up and going to a funny movie, usually alone. The date often begins from a sad state, where I wondered whether I could gather my energy to make it happen. Often I would jump in the shower, and try to sing "Splish, Splash," in an attempt to purge the tiredness, stress, and mental anguish. I could witness negative bubbles spiraling down the drain, and my off-key tones usually got me to snicker. Without fail, my huge shepherd dog, Puppy, always pushed open the bathroom door and tried to howl along in unison. This high-pitched yowling was a prehistoric remnant of some off-key, wolf ancestor.

One night after an incredibly harsh, ten-hour day, which included caring for victims of a subway collision, working overtime and understaffed, I dragged myself to see; A *Fish called Wanda*, starring John Cleese, Michael Palin, Kevin Kline, and Jamie Lee Curtis.

Driving myself to the theater, I inserted a tape of Woody Allen, doing stand-up comedy, as my humor warm-up. Settling into my seat at the theater, enjoying hot popcorn, I recovered from that horrendous day. "I've had it with hospitals," I thought. As if on cue, a man in a wheelchair silently rolled up to my isle seat and parked. Here I had come to court humor, and was soon dragged back to the *hospital view* of things! But a few handfuls of popcorn later, I noticed that for all his physical problems, the man had created his own good mood.

"I'm hooked on the *Flying Circus*," he volunteered, smilingly referring to the *Python* show starring John Cleese, and Michael Palin, from the BBC. "This is gonna be a treat." And it was. We were swept away by the madcap antics of bank robbers and barristers. We were treated to inane disguises, stupid food tricks, and yes, even funerals for dogs.

He had a relaxed sort of delight in being alive. He was in this mirthful moment, while I had been unable to shake off the day's trauma, expecting that the *Pythons* would do that for me. A handicapped man who had the gift of humor! His thoughts were close to joyful and thankfully they helped me to put a little more fun into the moment. Before the lights dimmed, we both laughed at the British way he could mimic John Cleese. *Releasing* the stress of the day led to good belly laughs, and those coaxed a comedic connection throughout my being.

This was a turning point. My worst workday stress, combined with bone-tiredness, had responded to being nursed back to health, by a team of comedians. I began a video collection. I couldn't know it was to be an invaluable means of self-treatment.

Laughing with Patients

▼

"It is through this language, the nonverbal language of laughter, that patients can speak the unspeakable and ask the unspoken questions. Humor becomes a way to communicate."

Colleen Gullickson, R.N.

Since the overworked nurses were often unreceptive, I zeroed in on another group, hungry for stress release: my patients. I resolved to have more fun at work. Thanks to my humor dates, and to meetings with the successor to Nurses For Laughter, the American Association for Therapeutic Humor, (AATH) my bag of tricks was getting bigger. I also got better at kidding around. One lady, who regularly needed help getting to the bathroom, became my dance partner. We would sing and hang onto each other, as we cha-cha-ed our way to the restroom. I also entered the very clownish world of props: gag items, toys, and stuff that had been time-tested in the circus. Props were usually successful, whereas jokes were a bigger risk. Though not interested in becoming one, I appreciated clowns, and hoped for a similar affect. I wished I could grab for a pair of Groucho glasses as easily as I dispensed Tylenol.

My early props were: a squeaker, a hammer and a five-pound aspirin. The squeaker was a plastic disk, such as clowns hide in their gloves. When they pinch a kid's nose, a mysterious high-pitched squeak escapes. The plastic hammer emitted the battery charged "crash," and tinkle of glass shattering. Then I shopped in Think BIG, a store full of oversized items, and came home with the five-pound aspirin. It was intended to be a paperweight, but I had other plans for it. As funny as the props were, my purpose was serious, as serious as my *designer wound dressings*. I *prescribed* carefully, a specific prop for the appropriate humor deficit, in a particular patient. At no time did I ever ask for anyone's permission to do this. Jokes, however, were often prefaced by, "Wanna hear a joke?"

At home one evening, I hid the squeaker in my white nurses' shoe, inserted my foot, and burst into hysterical laughter.

"You've finally gone off the deep end," my roommate, Ellen, sighed.

Recovering my breath, I replied thoughtfully, "This squeaks loud enough to echo through the hospital corridor." And then I knew the perfect application for this humor therapy.

I spent the better part of one workday trying to cut through Mr. Fred Frederick's negative energy. He refused to verbalize. He grunted or blurted out one word at a time.

"No." "Yes." "Good."

Fred's face was a mask, which appeared to have been frozen in the blizzard of '78. It never thawed. When a patient is unable or unwilling to participate in his care, it sets the staff toward a new series of obstacles, which usually slows down the patient's progress. His diabetic condition would respond to nutrition, medication and exercise, but communication was Fred's missing link. Without the process of communication, we staff members would need to rely on a significant other, in order to help him to use these tools.

At the close of my shift, writing in the chart about his depression, which was superimposed upon his medical problem; it occurred to me to use a prop, the squeaker.

On my morning rounds the next day, I entered Fred's room. I assessed his condition, I checked for the necessary supplies, and I made the usual, futile attempt at conversation. I made no reference to my shoes. They spoke for themselves. Fred's eyes darted toward the squeaking sounds, but he said nothing and remained frozen. I left the room and quickly retreated to the ladies room to laugh loudly before my lungs burst. I retired the device before continuing my rounds to the rooms of my other eight patients.

When Fred was due for his medication, I reinserted the squeaker in my shoe at the doorway of his room, and then breezed in as usual.

"Your shoe squeaks," Fred said, in a monotone.

I leaned closer to his face. His face seemed more animated, and it was as though the sound had struck a lost chord in his brain.

"I can tell you how to get rid of that squeak," he said, clearing his throat.

"You can?" I asked, innocently.

"Yes. Try rubbing saddle soap into the shoe leather." Fred's eyes had a new light behind them.

Hallelujah! Fred had spoken! There was a sense of ease within Fred's room. It was as though a storm cloud of pain had blown out the window of the sickroom. We had connected. I had managed to *squeak through*. A conversation ensued about his healthcare situation. The nurses on other shifts soon remarked about "a change in Fred." While his personality remained, the change was in his willingness to participate. Round two, going in with humor, had been worth all of the preparation, and effort.

I worked with Mr. Deseco, through a long string of admissions for eye surgery. The day that he planned to go home, his physician decided to do more tests, and cancelled his release. The patient was so angry that his blood pressure climbed above his normal reading. I listened as he vented his frustration, and then I excused myself from his room. When I returned, I found the man slowly, methodically punching his puny hospital pillow.

"Try this. It may be more effective," I urged, handing him the plastic hammer, which, when applied to his pillow emitted the sound of a picture window being shattered by a ball-peen hammer. When I passed through his room again, I heard him on the phone, feet propped up, telling his relatives that he was being held hostage in the hospital.

"Florence, my nurse here, gave me a...ha-ha-ha...a hammer to play with," he said, looking at and gripping the plastic handle hard, an unlikely weapon. "When the doc comes in tomorrow, if he holds up my discharge, I'll threaten'm with this," he promised, bringing the bogus hammer down on the receiver.

Crash! tinkle, tinkle, tinkle.

On the way home I felt that the hammer had been more effective to Mr. Deseco than any pill. A toy had given him a sense of control over his situation, and had left him relaxed. I remembered Sir William Ostler, a physician of the last century, who believed that a good doctor had to know how to distract the patient until his health returned.

The aspirin came in very handy. Annette, an elderly lady, and a delight to work with, never stopped smiling. That is, until her doctor started prescribing medication without notifying her or explaining its purpose. When I told her what the medicine was, its purpose, and the side effects, she thanked me, but went on to say that she was offended by being left out of her own healthcare.

I brought her the perfect antidote. Holding it behind my back, I said, "I've got a new pill for you, Annette. But this one you'll enjoy."

When she frowned, I passed her the *aspirin,* measuring six inches in diameter, and two inches thick.

"Oh wow! Now this is much better," she said, hefting the paperweight, "and it's the first pill that works by just looking at it! Will I be allowed to keep it 'til I see the doctor? I want to reprimand him, but I could *give* him your prescription at the same time!"

I went to work on Easter Sunday. The sun shone through my car window onto a newly acquired fuzzy headband, which supported white ears. At a stoplight, I slid it on my head, and looked into the rearview mirror. Above my auburn curls, I saw the white ears touch the roof of the car. Do I dare? I asked. I knew that if I did it, I'd have to do it today.

So I delivered all my patient's breakfast trays wearing a new sort of nurses cap. The kitchen had thoughtfully placed painted hardboiled eggs on each tray. The ears bobbed above my straight face. I was greeted first by double takes from the staff, but it was Deloris, a patient, who fueled my quest for humor with renewed vigor.

I slid the tray onto her over-the-bed table. She started giggling with a face I didn't know she could make. Her riotous laughing swept away my control, so that I had to lean against the wall, doubling over, laughing myself out of breath. It was a few minutes before we could speak. Alma, a nurse assistant, had come to see what all the commotion was about, saying over her shoulder, "Oh, it's Ditlow…" she sighed "up to her old tricks again," she winked, and moved on.

I stepped closer to the woman, who was being treated for a stubborn infection. Rigid infection controls had her worried about how long she would have to wait for healing.

"This is great," she said, still breathing heavily, "I needed this, stuck here on a holiday."

I asked her, "I have to know, Deloris, why do you think it's great?" By that time my fuzzy ears were on her head.

"Hee, hee, hee, oh that's simple," she smilingly choked, "It…it's the only thing in here that isn't sterile!"

Incongruity, yes, members of American Association for Therapeutic Humor had said that strangeness, weirdness and the oddities of life are often set ups for humor. A dignified man slips on a banana peel. The unsung quality of humor is that its good feeling usually goes beyond the humorous encounter. These examples of play with props connected others besides me, to the patient, other staff members, physicians, and family. Fred started to communicate. Mr. Deseco unleashed anger, and Deloris felt a release. The common denominator of all these humorous encounters, is that they ended with the sick person changed for the better, feeling better, *in better control of the situation.* Beyond humor, in each instance, the patient regained the control that is a part of being a whole person.

My humor campaign culminated in an all-out attack on the most ominous of patient stresses. Going to surgery. People going to the operating room are terrified of everything, from loss of their dentures, to death. I began by asking if the patient would be open to stress relieving techniques. In three years, I had only one refusal. Then I explained the pre-op procedure for that individual person. Knowing what to expect releases stress and reassures him. This completed, I diffused tension with the deep breathing techniques I learned in Yoga class. I was often sending people for eye surgery, and the eye drops blurred their vision. One of them disclosed that he feared his vision would stay blurred. I learned that deep breathing focuses the mind on the breath, coaxing tense muscles to relax as it infuses the body with additional oxygen. I could coach the patient while I did other routines; such as take the vital signs. If the workload was too heavy, I only had time for the above explanation, and to coach deep breathing, before the patient was whisked away. When that occurred, I felt that I had done my best to address and diffuse their fears.

Usually, time permitted part two of my stress relief program, which employed the patient's imagination. I asked the patient's help to *see* in his mind's eye, a safe, and successful journey through the surgical suite. This visualization was also useful because the relaxation it induced, tended to speed the effect of pre-operative sedation. Periodically, word filtered back from the anesthesiologist that the patient needed less sedation in the operating room.

When the call from the operating room came, I made it a point to be there to put the patient on the stretcher, to help her into her backless gown, and to tell a joke at the same time.

"You know why this is a gown made for the movies? It's rated *G* in front and *X* in the back!"

Having accomplished my professional obligations with the addition of humor, usually allowed the emotional needs of the patient to be addressed while I experienced job satisfaction. When post-op patients described how *easy* and *fast* their surgery was, I was gratified. Attempts at humor on my part were boomeranged back, and I, too, benefited from all the relaxation. My patients, who experienced it, showed a *team spirit*, and joked the next day as if we were friends. If my patients needed to be readmitted to the hospital, they often asked to be assigned to me. It was the supreme compliment.

Encouraged by my success, I wrote an article about nursing humor, published in *Imprint*, a journal for nursing students. At a trade show, I found a man who believed in the need for humor who produced corporate industrial videos. He helped me to make a short videotape about humor, as a tool for use at the hospital patient's bedside. Entitled *Humor Enhances Health*, I would promote it through nursing convention trade shows along with my humor presentations.

To make humor more widely available in hospitals, I created an interactive get-well card. I printed about thirty jokes on colorful strips of paper, and put them into plastic bags. When I decided to copyright the bag, I phoned my brother, Chris, who laughed, and said, "Call it Joke Poke." The *Joke Poke* became another way to have humor available in hospitals. People who bought my video would receive a *Joke Poke* as a bonus. I also handed them out to nurses attending my presentations.

I called contacts from the trade shows, and hospitals in the northeast to conduct humor sessions for nurses. By then I had observed that most women working in the hospitals have two jobs. They are responsible for the sick and injured for eight or ten hours a day, and then they return home, where they are responsible for the family. Constantly being on the giving, but rarely on the receiving end can unbalance the body, mind, and spirit. If unchecked, this situation leads to exhaustion, and total burnout.

The nurses attending my sessions needed a lift, but many just wanted to be passive, and wanted me to entertain them. What I wanted was for them to actively create ways to engage in humor regularly, so that burnout could be contained, and the energy in the hospital could have a chance to be positive.

To keep the group's, attention, I used props as *investigative medical instruments*. I chose as an assistant from the audience, a nurse with a back pain or a headache. I sought this nurse's funny bone-the humerus, by doing bogus eye exams. Juggling a plastic brain, I demonstrated brain balancing. I helped my assistant to open her chest by fitting her with a special humor vest. As I helped her don the vest, I chatted about the positive effect of hearty laughter on the cardiovascular system. Inducing belly laughs with the squeaker, and tapping an elbow to gauge its reflex with the glass shattering hammer, allowed the spirit to move, while I proposed my mission: infecting the hospital with humor.

> "Humor Interventions fit nicely into the third step of Alcoholics Anonymous (1976), which concerns itself with the concept of surrender and letting go."
>
> Donna Strickland

Genady and I decided we wanted to live together, and in 1991, I moved to New York City. I continued to do humor education sessions for nurses, but soon I would face a new audience, one with no good reason to laugh. I chanced to meet Burt Richterman, a homeless man on the F-train, in the subway car, while en route to a job interview.

He was yelling, "Buy humor! It's more powerful than Trump! It's more nutritious than Wheaties! More credible than Leona Helmsley!" He peddled his own cartoon paper, which used advertising to defray the cost of production.

In all of metropolitan New York, I managed to get on *his* train. Seeing that our missions were similar, and that he was about to leave the car, I had to make a split-second decision. Did I want to network with a homeless stranger? Yes.

I told him briefly about *Joke Poke*, and that I was new in town. He said that he had arranged humor meetings at a rehabilitation center for homeless veterans. He invited me to speak at his program for homeless vets. I accepted. Four sessions later, Ellen Carter, a social worker who directed the program for the Veteran's Administration, invited me to volunteer at the center on a weekly basis.

The Veteran's Administration treatment center was located on Seventh Avenue, at 24th Street. A variety of services were available: housing, financial support, counseling, and medical care. A security guard manned the door, and occasionally ejected veterans who attempted to attend the meeting while *under the influence*. The building had no windows, and inside, the paneling was dark. This should be a real test of humor therapy, I thought.

The center's director, Ellen Carter, informed me that the humor group would mostly be male, middle-aged, usually with medical problems, and lacking a supportive family. This was all the more reason to form a coherent, extended family, where no one was a stranger.

Later, when asked by a friend how I felt in a circle of drug and alcohol addicts, I rapidly answered, "Right at home!" I knew I had lots to learn from these veterans of war, about poverty, and hopelessness.

"I'm here because I can use a good laugh," I explained. I started by introducing myself, and revealing why, and how I came to the center. The veterans were not shy about expressing a need for humor, and they shared many examples. Our common ground was fertile for the establishment of a comfortable, safe, and trusting environment.

They were learning job skills, and making radical changes in an attempt to rebuild their lives. I wanted my humor to do its mind, and body magic, by releasing the stress encountered by homeless men, as they struggled to find housing, to get well, and perhaps to learn skills for work.

The weekly programs at the center metamorphosed from talking about humor in circles, to video showings. I brought many tapes, showing Eddie Murphy on *Saturday Night Live,* Lucille Ball in the candy factory with Ethel, the disrespected Rodney Dangerfield, and Gallagher, smashing watermelons. I used my prop play, as I had done with patients and nurses. I imported actors who were stand-up comedy students, and was lucky enough to have a visit from a pro, Steve Bhaerman, better known as: Swami Beyondananda.

I made an important observation after the first year. The veterans' body language, and verbal feedback told me that passive programs, that is, where I supplied all of the humor, were less effective than when the participants were actively involved.

Meetings where the members moved around guaranteed success. I knew the value of exercise in the alleviation of stress and depression, so I sought playful exercise suggestions from books written about the art of improvisation. New York is full of humor, and so supplied the perfect answer to the search for humor activity; improvisational comedy lessons for myself.

I spent three months at the Forty-Second Street location of the Gotham City Improv. From the very first lesson, I found the humor prescription for depression. I really sensed that therapy was happening for me in the release of my emotions, which improvisation requires. Improvisation doesn't ask us to be funny! However, it demands that we emote, that we say yes to the suggestions of the comedic team, and that we play together.

Two years after the veteran's group began meeting, I tested my newly acquired improvisation techniques with the homeless. When we worked as an imrov team, spontaneous smiles, and gales of laughter were generated. Unlike stand-up comedy, you were never standing alone. There was give and take, a pong for every ping, plus it took the pressure off me as the group leader. The unlimited comedic well of improvisation, allowed my groups to work hard, and to play effortlessly.

In 1987, I joined the American Association of Therapeutic Humor, (AATH) a group of believers who wished to apply the benefits of humor in healthcare. The group grew out of another group: Nurses for Laughter. Nurses, recreation therapists, psychologists, and doctors attend annual meetings where information is exchanged, and speakers can demonstrate their individual successes with humor.

Therapists of every description attended the annual convention: nurses, physicians, researchers, and clowns. We were united in our effort to infuse the lightness of humor into our hospitals, and into other humor-deprived institutions. The 1998 keynote speaker, Patch Adams, M.D., personifies humor therapy. He said, "I am more than a doctor, I am a clown."

Donna Strickland, R.N., is a nationally known speaker advocating humor as a component of health care. Speaking about the sound of laughter, she remarked that the sounds that we produce while laughing resonate, and clear the energy centers for major organs. The sound hee, according to Donna, vibrates through the head energy centers. Heh is associated with the throat, ha, with the heart, ho, with the solar plexus, and hoo is associated with the belly energy center. When I produced the manufactured laugh sound, "hee, hee, hee," I became lightheaded. I repeated, "hee," over and over, became out of breath, and then my real laughs took over.

"I'm empty headed," I gasped between laugh fits, vowing to spend even more time at this mindless activity. Other seminar attendees laughed along with us, getting our dose of humor simply by making the sounds "hee-heh-ha-ho-hoo." And importantly, getting it wholesale, without middle joke man!

Back at the homeless veteran's group, I reproduced these laughs that had welled up when I attended Donna's session on the sounds of laughter. Energy increased along with the laughs. I sensed that part of this energy was in the laughing voices alone. I considered how the voice quality of depressed people reflects their depression. A depressed person often masks anger at a situation, or at people, *including themselves*. Their voices are generally distantly apathetic as they struggle out of addiction. These are voices bereft of spirit.

"Who remembers a drill sergeant?" I asked the group as we stood in a circle.

This brought out smirks. Several heads bobbed up and down.

"How was the drill sergeant's voice quality?"

"Loud and demanding," someone replied.

I urged the use of this *in charge* voice with these energy laughs, saying; "Now *we* can be loud and demanding!"

"Hee."

"Hee, hee."

"Hee, hee, hee."

"Heh."

"Heh, heh."

"Heh, heh, heh."

"Ha, haa, *ha*!"

"Ho, ho."

"Hoo, hoo, hoo."

Soon they were laughing helplessly, and loudly enough that passersby poked their heads inside the doorway to see what was so funny. Even vets who described themselves as "having nothing to laugh about," or those who because of post traumatic stress syndrome or poor socialization, felt unable to laugh; began *cracking up.*

There were, of course, times during the ten years I worked with the homeless vets, that called for talk alone, times when we witnessed severe losses and intense emotion. Since therapy was my purpose and my goal, I addressed each meeting individually, which sometimes meant scrubbing the wacky program planned, in favor of a quiet expression of feelings.

In 1998, while I was grappling with my problems related to dental metals, faithful members of the AATH, Steve Wilson, a psychologist, Karen Buxman, an R.N., and Dr. Dale Anderson, an internist, went to India to witness and to learn about laughing groups, known as Laughter Club International. These groups sprang up in Mubai, India, in 1995, originated by Dr. Madan Kataria, a physician who felt that laughter groups could be offered to people in the parks. He combined the uplifting quality of laughter with the power of Yoga. After inducing laughter with jokes, and finding his repertoire depleted, he then decided to urge people to *laugh for no reason.* Necessity mothered a series of exercises whose goal was to keep the group laughing continuously for about fifteen minutes. The sequence starts with deep breaths, called, *Pranayama,* in Yoga. This is followed by frenetic clapping as they chant, "Ho, Ho, ha, ha, ha."

Participants greeted each other while laughing. Laughter is generated with the mouth closed, and then open, providing a good facial workout.

"The key is eye contact," Dr. Kataria told me, on his *World Laughter Tour.* It was the summer of 1999, and I made it a point to witness his exercise routine, with a group of enthusiastic office workers in Queens, New York.

"If you think I'm crazy for laughing for no reason," he told the group of a hundred, "and you laugh at me, then my mission is accomplished!"

If one hasn't actually laughed hard by this time, the next process, argument laughter, insures it. Dr. Kataria has a line of women, facing a line of men. They laugh while making eye contact and pointing their wagging index fingers at each other!

At the 1999 AATH convention, Steve Wilson presented his Indian travel-laugh-log, based on his visit to India. For thirty minutes, we conventioneers became a rendition of the Indian laughter club concept.

Despite my balance problem, I could do the exercises without difficulty, since the arms were more involved than the legs, and lungs more than the arms! In one exercise, we shook hands with other *laugh lovers,* while laughing as our arms pumped. Wow, I thought, would this be great to do with my group of veterans.

I returned to my humor groups of homeless veterans with an additional dose of laughter, thanks to the presentations of Steve Wilson. My session opens with an anecdote or joke. This allows me to sense the collective mood. I do different routines if it's an energetic group, as opposed to a group that tends to act more depressed.

Sometimes the depressive mood is so thick in the room, it's like sludge. Just getting out of his chair is an ordeal for one new member; another is distracted by sports pages. But one-by-one, they stand with me in a circle, doing Qi gong Chinese energy exercises to begin. This simple deep breathing combined with floating arm exercises could usually be counted on to open the eyes of the group.

The improvisation warm ups were usually capable of getting people moving, while making the group a team. Picture this: grown men tossing a basketball, and this ball is invisible. Invisible basketball became the cornerstone of my therapy. The eyes that were downcast now dance as they follow the ball. My strategy was to support the group effort by giving all of the participants a couple of turns with the *ball*, and then to maintain the momentum with other warm ups. *Clap, slap, snap* involved the unified group by clapping hands, slapping knees and snapping fingers *in unison*. I would insure laughs at the end with Indian Laughter Club style laughter as the grand finale. The entire assortment: anecdote, improv comedy warm up, and Indian style laughter, happens in one hour.

The plan for an energetic group was different, because they needed a bigger challenge. There were more and faster warm ups, which were followed by improvised sketches. The outcome often compared to the work of a professional troop of actors. Surprised by their own creativity, many veterans were amazed at having uncovered long dormant senses of humor.

"Eddie Murphy has nothing on you," I promised them.

Bill yells, "I sure could use Eddie's money."

"He is paid well and he practices," I reply. "He thinks about humor; he's learned how to be funny. But he started by believing in himself."

If there was a strong interest in improvisation, I continued with sketches, but usually I closed with a few Indian style laughs, and then signed off. A successful sketch was the *New York Party*. A volunteer was appointed to be the *host*. One-by-one, the other participants knocked on the invisible door, opened by the host. Each guest adopted the accent and mannerisms of a different ethnic group. The host tried to answer in the same manner, changing according to the guest.

Each week I reminded them, "Thank you for laughing with me. You have made my day." I was thanked and often hugged in return, by men who assured me that being in the group *felt great*.

My laugh therapy groups made everything go better for me, too. I scheduled doctor appointments after the laughs, so I could more easily endure the endless waiting for tests, the dental restoration, and my balancing act.

There was one session that did not conclude with the usual laughs. Instead we closed with a tear.

"I'd like to say something," said a staunch member of Comic Relief, clearing his throat. "Do you want to hear my favorite poem?"

We nodded affirmatively and got into our seats, while he stood, breathing deeply and dramatically began:

IF

If you can keep your head when all about you
Are losing theirs and blaming it on you,
If you can trust yourself when all men doubt you
But make allowance for their doubting too,
If you can wait and not be tired by waiting,
Or being lied about, don't deal in lies,
Or being hated, don't give way to hating,
And yet don't look too good, nor talk too wise:

If you can dream—and not make dreams your master,
If you can think—and not make thoughts your aim;
If you can meet with Triumph and Disaster
And treat those two impostors just the same;
If you can bear to hear the truth you've spoken
Twisted by knaves to make a trap for fools,
Or watch the things you gave your life to, broken,

And stoop and build 'em up with worn-out tools:
If you can make one heap of all your winnings
And risk it all on one turn of pitch-and-toss,
And lose, and start again at your beginnings
And never breathe a word about your loss;

If you can force your heart and nerve and sinew
To serve your turn long after they are gone,
And so hold on when there is nothing in you
Except the Will which says to them: "Hold on!"
If you can talk with crowds and keep your virtue,
Or walk with kings—nor lose the common touch,

If neither foes nor loving friends can hurt you;
If all men count with you, but none too much,
If you can fill the unforgiving minute
With sixty seconds' worth of distance run,
Yours is the Earth and everything that's in it,
And—which is more—you'll be a Man, my son!

    Rudyard Kipling

  I decided to give myself a year to prepare to leave my position as a psychiatric nurse, and to educate myself on the current ALS research. I subscribed to all the available ALS patient-centered newsletters, published by ALS treatment facilities. Month after month the newsletters arrived, usually with little in the way of treatment for the disease. I noticed a disheartening tendency in some of the articles that assumed their reading audience had one foot in the grave and the other foot on a banana peel. Skipping the pieces about impending doom, I decided to read the selections written by patients.

My favorite was by a man who walked into a research program for an evaluation. The therapist asked him to sit in a wheelchair and propel himself down the hall.

"But I don't *need* a wheelchair," he reasoned.

"Well, it's just on our list of activities for testing," she replied.

He saw the whole scene through the eyes of humor, which I appreciated, as I couldn't see value in assigning future weakness in the name of data gathering.

The worst-case scenario was inserted by researchers who wanted ALS patients to donate their bodies to their facility. "Sign for your autopsy in advance," it urged. Just the kind of news to cheer you up. It was hitting home with me, because I had just made a will. The words in the newsletter did little to encourage me. What I needed was to focus upon building up my belief in myself.

Besides the newsletter, I spent my free time that year reading a few books by professionals as well as patients with ALS. I was looking for strategies to guide me, a structure to work from, something positive. I didn't know how long I would live, but I was sure that I was not ready to sign up for an autopsy.

Gradually, I began to forgive the nincompoop. I decided that he did help after all, by sending me down a different path. He, more than anyone, had fueled my skepticism regarding allopathic medicine. Perhaps he was afraid that he would be held liable if he didn't give the implied poor prognosis.

I turned to Joe Adler, my chiropractor, who reminded me that contact with nature was therapeutic, and suggested that I regularly spend time outdoors. He also dragged a tome from the shelf, which catalogued hundreds of *spontaneous remissions,* and accounts of people with incurable diseases, who got well against all odds. I searched through the pages for recoveries from neurological disorders, and found a sole case of MS, which had mysteriously reversed.

He asked if I had considered an ALS support group and suggested, "Remember that some of the people there have been given negative messages, so they're likely to be filled with fear. If you choose to join them, don't identify with them."

He affirmed what I also felt about this. I decided not to go to the support group or to enter the research program. Instead, I chose a professional physical therapy office located inside of a health club. To me, physical therapy meant having an athletic coach. Mine was a tall, positive sort of guy, Scott Bedson, who focused my whole being on the functioning of my foot.

"Heel and push, heel and push." I listened to these words while walking on the treadmill, for forty minutes, every-other-week, for two years. Thousands of *heels and pushes* were performed. I did stretching, practiced balancing on a huge ball, and worked out on a multitude of weight machines.

Part of the therapy for me was that my coach always had a good story to tell. I listened to accounts of patients with neurological problems who had held on, and had refused to become discouraged. "Don't give in to spasticity," he warned.

Two years later, I left physical therapy to walk in my neighborhood or the local gym, balance on my own ball, and lift weights through water aerobics in the local pool.

One day as I was *heeling and pushing* slower than I would have liked, half way through a Union Square intersection, when a bus turned, in its inimitable New York way, blocking the traffic sign, which read: WALK.

The driver put on the breaks before running me over.

I yelled into the bus window, "It says WALK!"

"So walk," he replied blandly from above.

Finally! I had a body that could stop traffic.

I continued *heeling and pushing,* and arrived in the psychiatric unit of New York's, St. Vincent's Hospital, where I worked. Behind the locked door of our unit, lived persons in various stages of treatment for emotional and behavioral disorders. Thanks to these patients, I kept a grip on my own sanity.

As I entered this door, I was usually approached by a middle-aged woman with a clashingly, colorful outfit, and dramatic make-up. Her every word and deed indicated that she would remain hospitalized for the long term.

One day she wore a Hawaiian print dress, complemented by chunky sneakers, and tube socks. Her hair was medium length, and neatly combed. The ensemble would have been easier on the eye, if she had forgotten to wear make-up. Inside the unit door she greeted me. Her maroon lipstick and *pancakey* rouge were now about twelve inches away from my face.

"Hi, Florence, boy did I miss you," she exclaimed, rolling her eyes.

As I hung up my jacket, she gave an account of her day, which was touchingly punctuated by the gift of her newest poem:

I enjoy trees seen from the window
I love the clouds on high
The smell of grass soon to grow
SPRING!

The mentally insane helped me to appreciate my dire reality, and kept me from veering into hopelessness. Two patients suffered from an unusual eating disorder. They had the habit of eating dangerous objects. In the space of eight hours, one patient swallowed a fork, and the other had to be restrained from drinking water from the toilet.

Still, patients were often hardy from years of coping with a life unhinged from reality. Many were gifted in the arts and sometimes wisely philosophical. If these sick souls who had little education, and sometimes no source of income could learn to cope, then so could I.

I began conducting more humor support meetings at the hospital. Sometimes staff members joined and laughed with us. We were producing lots of laughs, most of them from joke telling. The following was my quick and easy recipe for a joke that yields belly laughs:

L: Light up when you tell your joke.
A: Animals never fail as subjects, for they have no religious or ethnic affiliation.
U: Underline key words. Underline means emphasize.
G: Get moving. Move your hands as punctuation.
H: Have one good joke memorized.

I believe that joking in a group is one of the truest forms of therapy. Learning that you are able to tell a joke can be uplifting for both you and for the group. People are always affected by jokes. Sometimes people love them, some hate them, and most say they enjoy hearing a joke. Usually people claim that they aren't able to remember any jokes. I feel that not remembering is a sign that the listener felt the humor and enjoyed the moment. If one decides to create humor by passing on a joke, recall is essential. Recalling a joke requires that a little effort be exerted. The joke must stay in your head longer than usual, and it will stay if you write it down. Retelling your joke will store it even longer.

Men will often say that their off-color jokes can't be told in a group where women are present. I have had to encourage them to tell their favorites in my presence, and I've never been shocked. Once told, a joke will trigger the memory of another joke, perhaps of a completely different type.

Joke School was intended for the humor of the moment, but with luck those dedicated souls who did their homework, would tell their favorite to a friend outside of the group.

I always reminded folks that we all have our own unique sense of humor. Following *joke school*, one of our *graduates,* a thin young man with a complexion the color of hot chocolate, offered to practice his joke. I felt that the joke he had memorized was priceless. Here it is:

One day the body parts were arguing. They had a difference of opinion as to who was in charge of the body. The brain said, "I think, therefore I'm in charge!"

The heart said loudly, "I'm at the center. I pump the blood. I'm in charge."

The hand said, "I handle everything. I'm in charge!"

"I'm the most specialized organ in the body. I move all the rest. I'm in charge," said the foot.

"I see! I'm in charge," said the eye.

"Oh, but I hear sound in the dark when you can't see," said the ear.

Before the other body parts could say anything, the asshole said calmly, "I'm in charge, and if you don't treat me with respect, I'll quit!"

Well, the heart and the brain laughed the loudest. They said, "Don't listen to him, he's only an asshole!"

Three days passed. Now the organs were very unhappy. The brain was unable to think, the heart skipped, the eye couldn't sleep, the ear was ringing, the hands and feet shook. Finally in unison, they begged, "Asshole, we'll respect you! Please be in charge!"

The moral of our story: an asshole is *always* in charge.

Nurses are given little in the way of humor education. This is unfortunate, because, as anyone who has endured illness can tell you, good humor is good medicine. Furthermore, when anyone shares humor, the effect is felt not only by the recipient but also the giver. Laughter, even smiling, changes communication. Humor and anxiety cannot coexist!

The value of smiling can be underestimated. A smile lends a sense of safety to a situation. Smiles are key tools for connecting through communication. Education, sales, or politics are indebted to the smile.

My early years in the nursing profession of the sixties were ultra professional. Large blocks of nursing education time were devoted to the conduct of the nurse, and very little time was spent on communication skills, which were largely relegated to the psychiatric specialty.

My patients were my best communication teachers. They have spoken to me deliriously in a fever, monotonously under the effects of anesthesia, and from the dark world of blindness.

Surgical discomfort didn't seem to be as painful as pre-surgical anxiety. Knowing how detrimental fear can be to the body, I was convinced that relieving anxiety could change a patient's personal outlook and pain quotient, for the better. I became more effective at expediting healing, and I began to see that sharing humor compassionately brings people into the present moment, safe from attendant fears. This fleetingly funny feeling is instrumental in creating a bond between patient and caregiver.

The joke above from the homeless man was priceless because it was funny, and funny partly due to the reality of constipation in hospitals. Constipation occurs simply because a patient's routine is disrupted in the hospital. As soon as I memorized the asshole joke, I was telling it to patients who came to me two times for a laxative. There was never a third request. I learned to cure constipation with humor! I became a walk-in joke exchange. Patients often came to hear my newest joke and often gave me one in return. I proved to myself that humor and laughing could affect the body in a positive way.

Throughout this period and especially during the early months of my illness, I often vented my frustration to Genady. A creative problem solver, at one point, he taught this subject to engineers. The basis of his course was the practice of concentrating on the problem, rather than on a poorly thought out solution. He has the gift of being able to think about a problem as though following the white line on the highway. He rarely loses his equilibrium, by veering onto the shoulder of worry, or by obsessive analysis. His genius is to be able to hold onto the moment, and to trust his own common sense. He seems to grow more intuitive as years pass.

His attitude toward my illness was, "Don't spend excessive amounts of time planning for a possible future problem, because if one does the proper work in the present, the problem may never come."

My lab results, which included a test for heavy metals, detected that the highest level of metal found was arsenic, and that was labeled: "within normal limits." "Where and when would I have been exposed to arsenic?" I wondered. It seemed less important to the doctor, than the other tests, and it *was* within the normal range.

I wanted to reclaim my health; I saw myself getting stronger in my mind's eye, my balance returning. I had even envisioned visiting the nincompoop.

What would I say to him? Thanks for jumpstarting me away from standard medical treatment for ALS. I decided to explore alternative methods to heal my damaged nerves.

1995: An End and a Beginning

▼

"Drive your own karma."

Swami Beyondananda

Dream…

Genady and I are riding in the backseat of my car, while being held hostage by two men: the nincompoop, and Dan Akroyd, who happened to be driving. Dressed as Beldar, the Conehead, from *Saturday Night Live*, Akroyd sits in the driver's seat, listening to the fuming neurologist's growls from the passenger seat, to "Drive!" The terrified Akroyd complies.

A screwdriver is stuck in the dash and I grab it, saying, "We can't be vandalized!" Meanwhile, the nincompoop eyes my pink handbag, which contains money, money that I will prevent him from taking.

Suddenly the two passengers in the front are out of the car. I stand up in the back and drive, as Genady notices the doctor, who is giving chase as we drive under a Long Island City elevated subway.

Interpretation: I am in the driver's seat. I will recover with Genady's help. I need more humor.

Dr. Chan did an EMG retest. My nerves were not reflecting ALS, she told me, but Primary Lateral Sclerosis.

She said, "ALS ravages muscles, which is not happening in your case. The nerve damage is somehow contained."

After six months of taking Riluzol, the drug designed to alleviate ALS, I stopped taking it. With the discontinuation of the drug, I had slightly more energy. I began to think about leaving my work in the hospital.

It was to be a gradual weaning from my job when something unexpected hastened my departure. A patient I will refer to as *Bob,* was in the hospital, and had been with us for two weeks. He was known for emotional volatility, and the inability to control his impulsive behavior.

He received medication for behaviors that included loud outbursts in the hallway, wrenching the phone away from a fellow patient, and for starting arguments in the TV room.

One summer evening, when things didn't go Bob's way, he plunged his fist through the wire-supported, glass window, of the nurses' station where I was working.

No one but Bob was harmed. Technicians accompanied him to the ER to suture a gash on his wrist. A housekeeper quickly swept up glass fragments before another self-destructive patient could hurt himself, or before someone could step on shards of broken window glass.

It was only later, at home that night, when delayed shock overtook me.

I said to Genady, "What if he hit someone?" I asked Genady, who was used to our *what if* games.

"What if he hit you?"

"I couldn't out-run him."

On any given day, this sort of problem could happen. I realized that the stress of working in a psych hospital in New York City, was taking a toll on my energy. Energy was in short supply, since the illness began. I did not want to continue to fray my already damaged nerves. I said a silent prayer of gratitude and decided my days at the hospital were at an end.

This decision was easy, but its ramifications were not. Starting at the beginning, I didn't know if I could live on Social Security Disability benefits. I did know, however, that the homemaker role held no appeal.

I picked up a book called the *Artist's Way,* by Julia Cameron. The book is an excellent resource for mental clarity through journaling. In order to find our creative selves, the author suggests we realize how addiction diverts energy away from time that could be spent creating something wonderful. While reading the chapter about addictions, I realized that I'm addicted to work! "*Hi*, I'm Florence, and I'm a workaholic."

It became even clearer to me when I stopped working. My family had provided my first job at the age of ten, at the place where I got hooked on work, Harrisburg, Pennsylvania. My relatives ran a bakery, which employed both of my parents. For removing empty breadboxes, and sticky metal pans from a local farmers market, my sister, my brothers, and I, were paid a total of ninety-one cents each, per weekend! You may wonder why not a whole dollar? In my aunt's opinion, it was more educational to pay a kid a penny, a nickel, a quarter, a dime, and a half-dollar.

Bakery work was harder than a stale cookie. My father surely violated the child labor laws by dragging the four of us to spend thick slices of our childhoods, immersed in the smell of birthday cakes, baking in the heat of summer, and winters cold enough to freeze egg custard.

My brothers, Chris and Jim, who assisted my father, worked the hardest and were treated to the grittier side of the place. They entered The Stitt Bakery: *the shop,* to insiders, at midnight; passing by giant sacks of flour, to enter through swinging doors, and into an oven-driven atmosphere where dough was king. The hard roll scented clouds hit them first, followed by the steam of chocolate cake batter, transforming into cup cakes, due to sell for five cents each. Turning into the heated section where cream-puff shells expanded, they were hit by a molasses haze that issued from the cookies that had recently been shoveled from pans almost as big as a small bed. The only quiet workspace waited for morning, when the cooled cakes would be artfully iced by Sarah and George, after all of the nighttime baking ceased, and when sugar seemed to precipitate from the air.

Chris and Jim made piecrust at an antiquated machine, which had a habit of groaning loudly, as though it had its roots in the netherworld. The pie machine stood on a wood floor, slick from drips of lard that accidentally spilled onto it. My uncle walked by with a long pole to which a scraper was attached. I recall that his scraping marches yielded burnt raisins, coconut, or bits of piecrust that had fallen off the worktable. The brothers sorted and piled into trucks, cardboard boxes of shiny chocolate-iced éclairs, glazed doughnuts, and cashew sprinkled breakfast rolls. These sugar-packed trucks then brought the goods to market by the time the sun rose.

Cindy, my sister, who was a *Jill* of all trades, was also famous for repairing the wobbly truck, which tended to *die* at traffic lights. She had the knack of being swift enough to do the repair, and then jump back into the truck before the light turned green. It's not a coincidence that she's now a nurse practitioner. She was a patient, unwavering, soothing influence on my father.

Daddy labored under the pain of arthritis. Work kept him mobile and gave him a sense of purpose, but it also drained him of any sense of pleasure or humor.

I was promoted to sales clerk at fourteen. The salary rose like yeast bread. That position in the sixties paid a whopping fifty-cents an hour! My early pattern was to be in school on weekdays, and to work on weekends. This basic scheduling of my work time, lasted until I graduated from the nursing education program, where the pay was only slightly better, and labor laws gave me two days a week off.

Recognizing now, that work had become an addiction, was an invaluable tool. Good health and a forgiving body allow overwork, but when I discovered I was a workaholic, I had to learn to rest deeply.

Judy, best friend since childhood, told me of the legend of Julian of Norwich. She presented me with a medal from St. Julian's home. The saint was a woman born in England during the middle ages, when people died young, and herbs were the only prescriptions available. Printed on the face of the medal was a saying attributed to Julian: All Shall Be Well, And All Shall Be Well, And All Manner Of Thing Shall Be Well.

Sickly Julian, in her monastery, expected to live out her last days. Apparently, she prayed so fervently for healing, that she recovered. Today, it is said that her strong spiritual presence lives on in the monastery.

I started praying to the God who wants me to regain my health. I bought a tape by Louise Hay, and listened to the expressions of love, which she's convinced, helped heal cancer. Her words wove themselves into my dreams.

"Deep at the center of my being there is an infinite well of love..."

Her technique for self-healing begins with thinking loving thoughts about oneself. She encourages the releasing of fear, describing it as an unwanted balloon on a string, which may be released. She reminds us that we are the only authority on our own life, and suggests practicing forgiveness.

How can I make healing happen, I asked myself, without a prescription? Make one up? Yeah, make one up. Now that I had left my work as a nurse, it was time to care for myself wisely. On a tip from my chiropractor, I began ordering detoxifying herbs by phone. The saleswoman asked for my credit card expiration date, which was 5/96. I waited for the transaction to go through and thought, "If the textbook at the neurologist's office was right, this card could outlive me. But I've got a lot 'a livin' to do," I thought, "I have to find a prescription." The herbal tinctures were designed to keep my body in an alkaline pH state. I would use these for nearly two years.

The search for the elusive prescription led me to my neighbor, Susan Singer, who had a doctorate in nutrition. My diet seemed to be adequate. She advised me to add several supplements to the ones I was taking, to insure optimal nutrition.

"Also, visualize yourself as well...imagine that you are already healed," she urged. Her recommendations were to take high quality multivitamins for nutritional balance. This would include:

Vitamin A, the vitamin famed for eye health, actually helps all tissue repairs. In addition to its many uses, it would be useful to a city dweller, for it protects against the ravages of polluted air.

B vitamins would act as insurance for optimal brain and nerve function. Other uses include cellular protective mechanisms and protection for the liver, which performs many functions, not the least of which is to detoxify.

Vitamin C, the esterified version, for immune enhancement and tissue repair.

Vitamin E, improves circulation, promotes healing, and helps reduce leg cramps. The use of it in combination with Vitamin C has a synergistic effect.

Coenzyme Q10 is an antioxidant, which increases tissue oxygenation, and is not adequately produced by the body as we age. It repairs tissue, notably gastrointestinal, cardiovascular, and gum tissue. Studies currently are underway, dispensing high dosages of this coenzyme to ALS patients.

Minerals:

The mineral calcium, not only builds bone and teeth, it aids muscular function, and the transmission of electrical and nerve impulses.

Magnesium assists calcium and potassium utilization and keeps the body pH in balance. It catalyzes enzyme activity, prevents muscle spasms and calms nerves. I was soon to discover I was low on magnesium, probably due to a compromised GI function. Most texts advise less magnesium intake than necessary for chronically ill persons.

Manganese also supports the nervous system, immune system, and blood sugar regulation.

Selenium offers glandular support to protect the immune system, and helps in the excretion of heavy metals.

Zinc works hand-in-hand with proteins toward anabolic activities such as wound healing. This simply means zinc will assist the building up of the body. I recalled elderly patients who had lost their senses of taste, and smell, but were able to restore them by supplementing a healthy diet with zinc.

Susan favored using flaxseed oil as a salad dressing, in order to get essential fatty acids. I was already taking acidophilus as a source of beneficial bacteria to support digestion, and digestive enzymes, to provide for optimal utilization of the foods I ate. While I cooked with garlic, I had never eaten it in large quantity, until now, in daily 1500 mg. oil capsules.

I was accustomed to getting nutrients from a balanced diet, but thought these supplements would insure that no missing links in the diet were forgotten. So, beginning with herbs and supplements, my holistic healing practices intensified. I talked about this with a friend who had once been my patient in the surgical hospital.

I remembered how Maria Tessier and I first met. She was sharing a hospital room with a woman who was having hourly panic attacks. This meant neither patient could rest. Medication did nothing to diminish the woman's anxiety. What did help were the calming suggestions of my friend. She assured her that we would not leave her, and urged her to breathe *into* the discomfort. I held the anxious woman's hand, while serving her a cup of hot tea. Maria had been through a more frightening medical situation than her roommate, yet summoned the strength to assist her. Later, as we related to each other as friends, she convinced me of the validity of visualization.

Based on her advice, I created an ideal scene in my mind. I saw myself riding a bike, laughing in the sun, a kind of *Clairol* commercial. I felt the pedals under my feet, the handle grips fitting my palms, and my sitting bones on the bike seat. I take in the view and hear humming as the tires meet the road. Genady rides between the river and me, and I stay perfectly balanced, on this tangible fantasy bike.

I told my friend Maria about my visualization. She shared with me that she works with her higher consciousness through spirit guides.

Maria said, "Spirit guides are, in a nutshell, intuitive thought, packaged as power persons. If you like, I'll ask for direction about your problem, and get suggestions from the guides."

Why not? I thought. The essence of the message from her guides was this:

"Honor the self."

"Take care of yourself first."

"A place inside needs recognition and healing. It's a place that was never nurtured. Allow it to emerge into the light."

"Recognize all feeling as good."

"Embrace feelings, and then release them."

"Ask your *own* spirit guides for direction, assistance, and above all, love."

"You are worthy of all your dreams and much joy lies ahead."

Well! That was promising. There was no mention of an immediate expiration date! The *place inside*, however, was a mystery. I supposed that related to my emotional health, which was important. The message at least verified that leaving hospital work had been a good move.

I remembered conjuring a couple of spirit guides after hearing a tape by Shakti Gawain, the author of *Creative Visualization*. She suggested to *just make-up* a guide. I decided on two guides.

They were anima, and animus: female, and male. The woman was a Native American elder, who wore a silky ceremonial dress. She was grounded and wise. Her male counterpart was Donny Osmond, filled with energy, dancing in a tux. When they worked together, his bow tie twitched with electrified energy, while her long dress billowed in the dessert wind. My team could produce guidance from the wisdom of the ages, and then had the energy required to put the wisdom into the ideal action.

I took time to tune into the guides while enjoying the park, the river view, or looking at clouds from a plane window. Tuning in to them worked well to assist in my everyday decision-making. They were reassuring, saying, "You're going to be OK," they insisted. "You're going to be OK."

A year had transpired since I retired from hospital work.

My balance was unsteady, there were occasional falls, but my speech was stronger. Not that I could speak at my former speed. I could not keep pace with the *fa-la-las*, while caroling at Christmastime, 1995. These sounds, that required an agile tongue, were incorporated into the visualization. The bicycling route could shift instantaneously to a winter scene. I was there, biking merrily over ice and snow, a figgy pudding in my basket! Genady sang, "Deck the halls!"

I sing my "Fa-la-la-la-la, la-la-la-la's."

What brought on the improvement? The herbs? The rest? The prayers? A heavenly host of angels? I had seen this force in the company of patients. The benevolent force came in the toughest times: when a surgical patient began bleeding, when a patient's pain did not respond to medication, and it pushed me to create a solution. Likewise, my own encounters with unbearably stressful moments had required that I stop, take a deep breath, and *know* that this force would see me through.

One day in early 1996, I asked God, the spirit guides, and the force, for help to call in this energy, in order to recover from my illness. A Tibetan monk was my answer.

My friend Joan, phoned, saying, "Yeshe Dhonden may be able to help you. He is a Tibetan Buddhist, who escaped from Tibet with the Dali Lama. Yeshe was his doctor, once upon a time. He's an herbalist, and hey, this guy looks like a mountain of a man."

I reflected, "A doctor who saved his own life, by escaping over the Himalayas. That is intriguing…OK, I'll check into it."

The respected man visited the States yearly, to work with an American woman, Marsha Woolf, also a monk, doing pulse diagnosis, urinalysis and prescribing herbal remedies. I took a cab to the office on west Twenty-third Street. A young man wearing shorts, a T-shirt, and Birkenstock sandals, opened the door to the office, and welcomed me to the waiting room.

I crept slowly to a seat near a photo of Dr. Dhonden. It had been taken as he walked with the Dali Lama.

Dr. Dhonden looked to be about sixty-five. Like all Buddhist monks, his head had been shaved. He was dressed in the traditional red robe. When I sat before him, he looked up from a Physician's Desk Reference? No, no, he was reading a fat, red prayer book. Once more my Western sensibility had collided with the wisdom of the East.

Through an interpreter, I told him I'd been diagnosed with ALS, and then Primary Lateral Sclerosis, that I was disturbed by unsteady balance, and a new symptom; muscle cramps. The cramps were likely to occur at night and were beginning to disrupt my sleep.

He took a minute to have me sit directly in front of him. He was not tall, not overweight, but Joan correctly saw that he resembled a mountain. Pressing against the radial bone of my right wrist, he took several pulses, and then moved to repeat the process on the left.

The doctor took my urine to an outside patio, to do his analysis in the sunlight. I was curious about the analysis. The interpreter only said that the odor, and the color were taken into account. Meanwhile, I noticed the *pharmacist*. Dressed as a monk, he said nothing, as he worked feverishly, placing little balls of herbal remedies into plastic bags, under the gaze of a large statue of Buddha. On the floor, near a huge gold urn filled with flowers, a lounging, husky dog wagged its tail against the floor.

Without having seen me walk, the Lama remarked through the translator, that he supposed my gait was uncoordinated. He described the way that my heel struck the ground, wobbling before pushing for the next step. His years of pulse taking and urine diagnosis had led him to this astute conclusion.

My understanding of Tibetan medicine is that it relates to the Earth. All living things are composed of earthly elements: earth, water, fire, air, and space. Dr. Dhonden determined that the air element was the problem. He would suggest dietary changes and herbs. There were at least twelve different herbs from India, but the translation of them was difficult. I was assured that they had no side effects, and to write to India for refills.

I left with four small bags of the marble-like herbal pills, and herbs, including a mysterious precious herb, which was a combination of the different varieties, wrapped in pink silk. The doctor himself tied these with multicolored strings, while he prayed for the one who would consume the pill. Precious herbs bore the physician's insignia in an orange stamp of wax.

He suggested a diet that eliminated coffee, alcohol, pork, watermelon, pineapple, and carrots from my intake. The interpreter told me that a woman, who had been bed-ridden with a similar complaint, had become mobile after following this same prescription.

"Why not carrots?" I wondered later that evening, as I made vegetable soup minus carrots. I thought over my meeting with the Tibetan Lama. I felt that taking additional herbs did not pose much of a risk, and I could easily adhere to his dietary suggestions.

I was moved by the contrast between Dr. Dhonden's office, and the neurologist's office. Both had their big city following, and both had a seriously ill clientele. The neurologist was so disconnected from me, the patient, that his very presence drained me. The Lama's surroundings were filled with love; imagine, a friendly dog in the office!

I would chew the herbs religiously, for nearly four years, at a cost of thirty dollars a month. They appeared to look like innocent chocolate drops, but tasted like aspirin. Within the first month, the cramps lessened considerably, but my balance continued to be precarious.

The physical therapy, P.T., strengthened my muscles, but was not helping my balance. Returning from P.T., I got off the bus near a community bulletin board. A sign read: "T'ai Chi," with Jamie Guan, instructor. All in one day, I was going to go from Tibetan medicine to investigate Chinese martial arts.

I had heard about Jamie, but that was due to his fame as the choreographer for the Peking Opera. He had done the choreography for the movie, *M. Butterfly*.

Twelve postures were demonstrated over the next three months. I concentrated on the positioning of my body, inviting the chi to take off. I so needed a blast of energy to help me cope with persistent falls.

Near the East River, I began meeting weekly in a small group session. Jamie was living proof that daily consistent practice builds energy. He too, was a mountain of a man.

There was a thin, soft-spoken woman, named Barbara Ostland, who was in the class. We became friends while practicing *holding the tree*, one of the many exercises.

Jamie coached, "The feet should be standing under the shoulder. The shoulder relaxes. The hands face each other, not touching. Move your hands in and out. Breathe deep. Focus on the tan tien and think about yourself."

The meditative postures definitely moved the chi. Calm moved in with the morning breeze. Tan tien referred us to the area around the navel, a crucial location for martial artists, or for people interested in achieving a balanced posture.

While approaching the more complex stances, Barbara and I often looked at each other, puzzled, when the hand movements just didn't seem to go with the foot movements. Time and again we would encounter the same problems.

"I feel that the connection is lost between the movements," I said.

Barbara replied, "I just can't seem to make any progress."

After class we took our frustrations to the instructor.

"I can't remember the forms," Barbara said.

"Do you practice?" he asked.

"I started, but I soon stopped because I don't feel I do the right moves."

"If I learned each form, like a dance step," I interjected, "I think I'd remember the sequence."

Jamie promised, "I'll bring some sketches of the forms next time."

What a difference a sketch made. In no time, Barbara and I were doing the twelve forms with fluidity. I was balancing slightly better following the practice, which would be a good habit for the next two years. T'ai Chi not only helped the balance problem, it was also my introduction to the study of energy as medicine.

I practiced T'ai Chi routines for two years, and finally stopped needing a class. I ran into Barbara, as she was race-walking in the neighborhood. We sat for a while under my favorite tree. With its gnarly web of roots, one must search for a spot to sit comfortably under its sheltering branches.

She shared news about her grandchild and family that day, and we laughed over our progress with T'ai Chi. It seemed ironic that we couldn't get it while watching demonstrations, but we became masters when we saw sketches.

She asked, "Do you think your health is improving?"

"I'm kind of confused at times," I related. "My voice is clearer and I have less trouble talking, but my balance…ahh…well, I'm trying different things, now that I have a little more time. My next appointment is with an M.D., who practices Ayurveda. I know from Yoga practice, that Ayurveda is concerned with natural healing practices."

"Isn't that an ancient Indian form of healing?"

"Oh, are you familiar with it?"

"I just read an article somewhere about Eastern practices for long-term healing."

I asked her what she thought about such practices.

She thoughtfully answered, "Those ancient cultures see that health is time-honored, a lifestyle, not a pill or a short stay in a hospital."

1995 Continued

▼

Ear: My ears drain a clear fluid, about every other day.

Nose: In cool outdoor temperatures, my nose drips like a faucet from October to March. The year round violent sneezing episodes. I can sneeze furniture across a room.

Throat: Voice has improved projection this year. Speech slow, and occasionally slurred, hypersalivation. Not so easy to talk around this amount of saliva. Gum disease. Some soreness and pockets around a few teeth. Difficulty swallowing liquids and swallowing medicine in the form of large pills.

Cardiovascular: Low blood pressure, low body temperature, my feet are so cold in winter that Genady screams if I touch my feet to his, in bed.

Neuromuscular: Lack of coordination and balance. Walking is precarious. Spastic muscle movements. I lose my balance turning on the kitchen faucet or opening the refrigerator. Cramping muscles, especially at night and in calf muscles. Due to cramps, sleep is interrupted. At risk for falling: what an understatement! I needed a cane.

Emotion: Fear of going out in bad weather due to poor balance. Am I agoraphobic? Energy inconsistent.

My symptoms flashed through my mind as I walked to my Ayurvedic appointment. *Ayur* in Sanskrit, means science of daily living, while *veda*, denotes knowing. The doctor is an American, who graduated from medical school in India, and has for many years, practiced Ayurveda. I envisioned myself accompanied by the ancient Indian woman and the tuxedoed Donny Osmond, *Harvey-like* creatures, invisible to all but me.

They would look out for me, and prevent me from choosing another misguided nincompoop.

The door, wooden with a heavy glass window, weighed more than I did. The huge door pressed against elbow and ribs as I became wedged between it and the frame. I had lost about ten pounds since quitting my job. Pushing out would risk a fall. The amiable secretary freed me, ushering me into the small, lavender scented waiting room, and then to the basement office.

The site of his office in Greenwich Village, on a brownstone-lined street, was a familiar place to me. The hospital in which I had worked was just a few blocks away.

We introduced ourselves. His name was Scott Gerson. While he reviewed those tests done for neurological diagnosis, I saw that his desk was decorated with a vase of daisies, several chunks of amethyst, and a stainless steel thermos. Fish did their *finny* thing in a neon lit tank by the wall.

"Please, call me Scott."

He must have seen me admiring his oriental rug. He remembered finding this carpet in India, on one of his trips while finishing his Ph.D., in Ayurvedic medicine.

"I'm pleased to meet you, and how did you learn about me?" he asked after he reviewed my tests.

I told him that I'd seen his book on Ayurveda, in Barnes and Noble, and that I wanted to practice it. I said that I had stopped working and wanted to nurse myself back to health.

"Western medicine is based on *science*," he replied. "Ayurveda is also a science, but based on balancing body, mind, and spirit, instead of treating symptoms of illness, as we do in the West. Ayurveda is also a philosophy, one which seeks to achieve balance by coordinating our lives with the cycles of nature." He glanced at my tests and cocked an eyebrow. "I see you're an R.N., and you're interested in alternative healing methods?" he questioned.

"As a matter of fact, I just returned from the annual meeting of my professional organization, the AHNA; American Holistic Nurses Association."

It turned out that he was a member of the AH*M*A: American Holistic *Medical* Association. The meeting I attended had convened the AHMA, and the AHNA, at the same location.

"Did you explore any of the holistic treatments they offer at the meeting?" he asked.

"Three sessions, all of which I found powerful: Healing Touch, Transformational Breathing, and Body Memory." Each of these works by opening energy pathways through the body, which helps the body to heal itself.

"The thing that I needed most was to cry," I admitted, "because I sure went through the Kleenex."

"It was probably a good cry," he said, while doing the Ayurvedic version of pulse diagnosis.

Laugh and the whole world laughs with you. Cry and you look like shit, I remembered a patient once said, while Scott diagnosed my pulses.

His pulse assessment was similar to Dr. Dhonden's. He waited until I had been sitting in a chair for at least ten minutes. Then he found the locations on my wrist, which related to the three earthly elements: fire, water, and air.

All living things reflect the elements of the Earth, which are fire, water, earth, air, and space. The pulses reflect these elements. The pulse assessment shows one what elements are imbalanced. It also indicates the patient's body type, or dosha, which enables the practitioner to offer balancing herbs and therapies.

While the doctor assessed my pulses, I drifted back to the recent energy sessions at the AHNA meeting. I had managed to open the lid on the package of fear that the neurologist had handed me. I thought at the beginning of the first session that it was appropriate to be shaken by a life threatening illness. By the time the third tear-filled session ended, it brought back the words of Maria, my friend. I remembered her words: "A place that was never nurtured needs recognition and healing." In that place was my father.

My father was a loving and strong person, until pain from arthritis ground down his self-confidence. The pain bred a destructive fear; fear of not being a good provider, and of eventually not being capable of working.

Moving through this pain, which affected most of the joints in his body, he worked a six-day week, and did upkeep as well as additions onto our house. I remembered that he visited a doctor who gave him the then popular gold injections to relieve the arthritis. Instead, the *metal* caused a life-threatening episode of kidney failure. But his miraculous recovery did not change his work habit.

"You kids have it easy," he'd say. "What if you had to feed hogs? Kill chickens? What if you had to clean a cider mill?" The farm also pressed apple cider for surrounding farms.

He often reminisced about the actual workhorses of his youth. He identified with them. He was himself a workhorse, before husband, before father, before friend. As he became less able to work, he began to *use* his children for assistance, not as abuse, but unconsciously, as if we were appendages, helping to continue his momentum. After all, work was necessary, and a good thing.

By the time I became a teenage bakery clerk, he seemed to think less of himself. His worry grew into a cold, stagnant, cocoon. This could have been clinical depression, but we will never know. He began relating differently when I was eleven, and posing a question to him was often a lost cause. Rather than have a discussion, he was likely to make a judgmental statement or to detour off the subject. In many of my attempts to converse with him, my message wasn't received. Messages from him to me were always about work! Home from school meant an opportunity to work, never a conversation.

Everything about him changed, and as a child laborer of eleven, I took it personally. It was difficult to be in the same room with my father, and I avoided him after a while.

I stumbled into the unrecognized, unhealed place: his illness, which was interwoven with mine.

The therapeutic sessions at AHNA were ideal. The Healing Touch session was a form of therapeutic touch. During this session, I cried constantly, for half an hour. Tears surfaced that had been leftover from the shock of the diagnosis, and others spilled, like a waterfall from my soul. It felt good.

Transformational Breath involved deep breathing while receiving prompting by therapist, Judith Tache. Oxygen infused rapidly, in waves that resembled the conscious breathing of meditation, yet, it was so much more. I experienced what I can only guess was an out-of-body experience, in which colors pleasantly glowed. After the session had progressed for half an hour, the therapist suggested I slow down the deepest breathing. The accompanying feeling of suspended animation prepared me for her question: "Who is in the room?"

Without thinking but without a doubt, I replied, "My father."

She continued, "He's concerned for you. Tell him it's OK for him to go into the light."

"I'm fine, Daddy. You can go into the light," I answered slowly, while thinking, wait a minute, he has been in that light for years.

Finally, I decided to do a uniquely powerful session called Body Memory. This was a potpourri of energetic healing techniques. Doug Norment skillfully combined prayer, Reiki and color therapy. Reiki is another type of gentle hands-on healing. Due to the priming of the previous sessions, I was ready to go for the gold.

Opening with prayer, the therapist asked me to attempt to imagine colors moving from foot to head. These were colors of the light spectrum, which related to the basic human energy centers, or Chakras. We all have these energy centers, which correspond to major organ systems in the body. One-by-one, I moved red, orange, yellow, green, and blue. Then I stopped. I could not move the color indigo, a dark blue.

"Where does the color stop?" asked the memory therapist.

"At my knee."

As I received Reiki, I recalled that day when I first feared for my father's safety.

"I was five. He had been involved in an accident with the bakery truck, which resulted in a knee injury. The wide, shiny scar looked painful," I explained to the healer.

As I began shedding tears, the color indigo moved, stopping at my elbow.

I *saw* a broom, my own hand, and again, crying wrung the memory from my subconscious.

"I was around fifteen, coming home from high school. I met my father as I came in the kitchen door, but he didn't greet me. He asked me to sweep the driveway! He wanted us to do his work," I excitedly explained to the therapist. I had never enjoyed crying so much in my entire life.

"Would you try to walk in a line, heel to toe?" Scott asked.

Returning to the present, I started to walk across the room. I took about five steps, and then veered from the imaginary line, unable to keep my balance.

When I sat down again, he said, "There are many diseases which can be healed to a large degree, by Ayurveda. I think yours may be one of them. One thing I'm always encouraged by is the tendency of allopathic physicians to change the diagnosis as the patient improves; and they changed yours from ALS to Primary Lateral Sclerosis."

"When you took my pulses, what did they tell you?" I asked him.

While answering, he drew a diagram. "Not only are you walking off balance, your body is Ayurvedically unbalanced. This is partially because of Western mans' tendency to go against nature, instead of with it. The simple answer is that your vata element needs to be pacified, and your pitta element needs support. You'll see what I mean as you try my suggestions." His diagram showed a horizontal line, representing normal. Kapha was on the line, but vata was up, as if shot from a cannon, while my pitta element was sluggishly down in the cellar.

He closed the session by adding, "Your body type is vata-pitta."

I was given a list of handwritten instructions. He urged me to meditate, do Yoga, and spend time outside in sunny weather. His assistant, Fredericka, put some intriguing items in a brown paper bag, then explained what to do with them.

The fall and winter period, vata season, as she had described it, was just beginning. The Manhattan evening had a chill in the air. She told me that the same cool vata quality in nature resides within human beings. The items she had in the paper bag would strengthen my body by balancing vata and pitta, which were two of the three doshas.

According to Ayurveda, everyone has qualities of the three body types; vata, pitta and kapha, but usually, we are influenced by two dominant doshas.

Vata types are usually short or thin, tend toward over exertion, moving and talking rapidly. Like winter, they are identified by dryness. These people have dry hair, cool, dry skin, and scant perspiration.

Pitta types have well-proportioned bodies, and rarely miss a meal. Like summer, they tend to be fiery in temperament.

Kapha types are large boned, and have tendencies for weight gain. Their calmness and slow pace provides for excellent stamina. Like spring, they have a watery quality and may tend to retain water.

This was my initial understanding of the way Ayurveda sees our bodies. Fredericka suggested that I drink about a cup of plain hot water hourly, during the day hours, to counteract dryness associated with vata, and to promote digestion. I would also make a tea from fresh ginger. Maybe ginger is a lifesaver. I grew to like this root for its warming properties, such as soothing indigestion, and easing muscle cramps. It even has antioxidant activities in the body. Later I would be juicing raw ginger root.

Daily self massage with sesame oil was recommended and demonstrated. I would do that prior to bathing so the circulation would be enhanced, speeding removal of toxins. Massage is friction, so it heats the tissues and stimulates nerves.

In a small aromatherapy cup, she demonstrated how to heat lavender oil by the fire of a candle. The doctor recommended I begin with lavender, queen of the oils. Calmed nerves were insured by the oil, which would affect neurons in the brain via my olfactory nerves. In addition, I was to place hot packs on the abdomen weekly. The packs would help digestion and clear the toxins present in the liver.

Finally, Fredericka handed me a sheet of dietary guidelines. "Eat warm winter foods, like root vegetables; sweet potatoes, squash, and beets. These will be nurturing for your vata energy," she advised.

The Ayurvedic diet that she had recommended was unusual in that very few foods were off limits. Refined sugar and coffee were out, but what was in was a wide variety of food choices. Scott advocated smaller amounts of food per meal, to help stoke a *digestive fire*, the better to burn calories, by leaving room in the stomach after a meal for space and water. Scott and his assistant had spent more than an hour with me, the lengthiest doctor visit I had ever recalled having. What's more, I could continue my multiple supplement and Tibetan herb routine. The diet would remove sugar once and for all, and reduce the use of bread, adding whole grains. The net result was a ten-pound weight loss in two weeks. I believe the deleted sugar accounted for the weight loss.

The therapies outlined to me were certainly affordable, I thought, but they required dedication. I did not take naps easily. The vata element provided a life centered on motion and change. Now, in it's current state of imbalance, I was more aware of chronic exhaustion. Building the pitta element helped my digestion and pushed me to take on the illness more aggressively.

After two months of conscientious Ayurvedic practices, I returned to the office. Scott was pleased by the progress I had made, though my balance remained uncertain. He suggested that I think about *winter hibernation* for the purpose of calming vata. I recalled again the advice of Maria's guides: *honor the self.*

1996

▼

The year 1995 ended, taking a large blanket of my fear with it. I had seen how much was possible through intention, and joining forces with nature. My self-prescription involved a vegan, vegetarian diet, including nutritional supplements. The list of my regular practices included:

Tibetan herbs
Meditation
T'ai chi: three times weekly
Ayurvedic self massage, hydration and enemas
Visualization
Acupressure
Humor

Calm began to set in as I decided to go organic. If I had come this far in improving my health, then I did not want to waste my time by ingesting sprayed chemicals and nutrient poor produce.

It also made sense to use seasonal produce. Without a nearby health food store, how would I carry heavy grocery bags? The lightweight of a briefcase was enough to unbalance me. These problems were solved one autumn day as I steamed yams, listening to the audience-supported New York radio station: WBAI, 99.5. Shelton Walden of "Walden's Pond" was interviewing a representative of an organic produce company.

Had I heard correctly? Could groceries be fresh, organic *and* delivered? I quickly dialed Urban Organic's 800 number. A few days later, I received three boxes of choice organics. They provided the produce, plus an assortment including fresh basil, eggs, orange juice, bread, chilli, olive oil, and even chocolate pudding.

Freedom from grocery shopping was mine! I ordered just enough prepared soups, lasagnas, and veggie burgers to avoid family grocery shopping, and standing in the check out line. I felt great about supporting a company that helped save me so much time and energy.

Soon afterward, serendipitously, another radio announcer, John Harris, interviewed the author of an Ayurvedic text on the subject of doshas. I tuned in at mid-interview, while I seasoned my rice with red pepper. Adding turmeric, it magically turned yellow.

"Doshas are referred to in Ayurveda as bodily humors. The three doshas are; vata, pitta, and kapha. Everyone's body is composed of all of these elements, just as the earth is."

"Vata, a dry, cold dosha, which is linked to movement, likes warm foods. Pitta, a hot dosha, associated with the heart, responds to cool foods. Kapha, a dosha, governed by water, associated with the head, is balanced by light, stimulating foods."

The speaker went on to say that imbalances usually manifest themselves as an exaggeration of our usual tendencies. A vata imbalance could be aggravated by the energy of the cities fast pace, going without rest, even long phone conversations. The author emphasized that one could practice Ayurvedic healing methods without being an expert on the subject.

This news was very encouraging to me, in my already compromised state. I was beginning to wonder whether I possessed the mental and physical moxie to pull the whole thing off.

The announcer questioned his guest about her ideal Ayurvedic day. She gave the following schedule:

6-7 A.M., Arise and drink hot tea
Eliminate
Perform Yoga or walk

Meditate
7-8 AM, Breakfast including hot drinks throughout the morning, water being the preferred choice
Follow with work activities.
12-1 P.M., Lunch to be consumed enjoyably
Short walk for optimal digestion
4 P.M., Tea break
Rest or meditate in early evening
6 P.M., Evening Meal
Short walk for optimal digestion
Satsang: Evening spent with family or friends, usually a humor filled encounter
10 P.M., Bedtime

Modern scientific research substantiates the healing power of Ayurvedic medicine. Herbal combinations, Yoga, rest, and complementary diet for the body type are the mainstays of the practice.

She also mentioned a means of Ayurvedic detoxification, a sort of ritual cleansing called Panchakarma, used as a means of removing the cause of disease. I was to become intimately acquainted with this *jewel of Ayurveda*, but at that radio minute, I didn't pay it much attention. I was wondering how I might adjust my schedule to arise at dawn, and what about going to sleep at ten P.M.? It had been a difficult change, to go from nurse to patient, but I had made a beginning. Thanks to the medical data on the radio, I felt like the call letters could be w-HOPE. Hope was on the horizon and gratitude grew within my heart.

New York City: The only place in the world where you can be deliberately run down by a pedestrian.

Florence's favorite ways to describe falling down, with apologies to David Letterman:
Hugged the ground

Stopped, and got instantly horizontal
Got Gravel faced
Saw the sidewalk up-close
Went to Ouchland
Went to the concrete chiropractor
Slid off the wall
Did the banana trick
A graphic demonstration of the law of gravity
Passed the osteoporosis test
Fell off the horse

One warm spring day, as I was slowly proceeding from the subway, with a cane, in order to meet some friends from England for tea, I felt it begin to rain. My creeping pace convinced me to take a cab, although they are usually scarce in bad weather. I inched off the curb, stood in front of a car parked at Sixty-Third and Lexington Avenue, braced myself on the cane, and stuck out my other arm.

Rain pelted my baseball hat for what seemed like a very long time, when a yellow cab stopped, ten feet away at a red light. I moved towards it at my snail's pace. A woman with a briefcase, coming from the opposite direction, jumped in the backseat. My moan of disappointment was lost in the patter of rain and the din of traffic. I started to wish I'd walked, but I leaned on the cane, and raised my arm in the air.

After ten minutes another cab pulled up, only to be snatched by a man who pretended not to see me. The next thing I knew, an impatient, dark, handsome man, was standing over me asking if he could help me up.

When I realized he had bowled me over from behind, I wanted to strike him dead with my wet cane. Instead, I burst into tears. A woman witnessing the scene came rushing over.

"I saw you knock her down!" She vituperated against my would-be assailant.

"I'm trying to help," he explained.

Meanwhile, having gotten to my hands and knees, I regained my footing. "Are you OK?" they both asked.

"I'm not crying because I fell," I sobbed between sniffs, "I'm crying because...because...I can't get a cab! I've been waiting here for an hour!"

Neither had an answer to this singularly New York curse, and in their impotence, quickly disappeared. As luck would have it, a cab appeared just as the rain dispersed. In my bedraggled, mentally altered state, I assumed this yellow box on wheels was a mirage.

It whisked me to my rendezvous with my English friends, Val and Anne, where I enjoyed the best cup of tea I ever had, explaining the reason for my disheveled appearance. My friends agreed that their shopping spree in chaotic Times Square was much less of a hazard than my search for a cab in the rain.

Falling was a scary proposition; the unpredictable loss of balance coupled with the possibility of injury.

What is worse than bruises, cuts, and struggling to my feet, is the shock. Traumatic shock is the state brought on by the jarring of the physical frame, coupled with adrenalin-powered anxiety.

I typically caught my breath, checked for obvious injuries and then slowly got to my feet, usually with a cane if I was alone. Trauma also may bring with it an energetic shift whereby the human energy field surrounding the body is torn or misaligned. Because of my precarious balance, my physical therapy coach had suggested that I read a good book on balance exercises, *How to Prevent Falls*, by Betty Perkins-Carpenter. I was now in the habit of doing my therapist's favorite balancing exercise on a large blue ball, two feet in diameter. This was further insurance, though no guarantee that I would not fall in the future. This gigantic ball was the most recent addition to my collection of health promoting materiel. I had already bought myself a cane. I wore only flat oxfords with bump toes, and though not fall-proof, the turned up toe avoided tripping. I had removed all carpets in my home, as my footing is surer on bare floors.

Outside my home, the ever-present danger of potential injury awaited me. I have fallen when the subway train lurched. I've dived head first in the subway station. I've landed in the sand on vacation, fallen in a public bathroom stall, while trying to flush the toilet with the cane, upended myself on my mother's plush rug, tripped into an elevator, keeled over in class at a conference and I have even been knocked over by two small boys and one large unsaintly Saint Bernard.

During these years when I awarded myself a gold medal in the category: *falling on the ground*, I made a discovery. Babies are the true experts in this category. In my opinion, toddlers see falling as just an interruption in their daily activities. First, they display surprise. They often cry, but not for long. What is good about toddlers is that they don't obsess about the unpleasant falling episode. Never embarrassed, they forget about it and amble away, to yet another adventure.

Following my fall in the rain, it became clear to me that mobility is the natural manifestation of my vata nature. Mobility, like eating, is primary. I vowed to be true to my mobility, even if that meant falling, when it was least expected.

The immediate benefit of a cane is that people notice that you need a little more room, and will often give you a wider berth. In New York, the pace is fast, but despite the rush of this city's life, people have the lovely habit of holding the door for the next person, especially if you happen to have a cane. I discovered that canes have uses other than as walking sticks. I can stop elevator doors from banging shut by waving it in front of the electric eye. With cane-extended arm, I have pulled an earring from under the table, turned off a light, and pulled a bag of spaghetti off the top kitchen shelf.

Speaking of falling and canes, what about falling *with* a cane? One cold and rainy night, I did just that. I'm grateful that this pitiful mishap occurred in the company of my friend, Ellen. Otherwise, consequences could have been dire. We walked arm in arm, Ellen was on my left, while in my right hand I held the cane, to help to keep my balance.

Suddenly, I passed the *osteoporosis test*. Sitting on the wet pavement, I searched for a reason for the fall. I hadn't tripped, nor seen a hole in the sidewalk. Then I erupted in a choking laugh spasm. Naturally enough, my friend mistook it for crying.

"Look!" I gasped, holding up my aluminum cane in the foggy night mist.

"Wow," Ellen replied, "How'd that happen?"

My aluminum cane was now the shape of a dog's leg.

A passing neighbor, seeing this sight, said he thought it was about as funny as a rubber crutch. An ice pack soothed my bruised bottom, but not my firm resolve. The next day I wrote the following letter:

Dear Customer Service:

I am writing to inform you of an unusual occurrence connected with an adjustable aluminum cane (#number). I purchased this cane three years ago. On January 22, while walking in the street with a friend, the cane broke in the center, causing me to fall.

Thanks to my friend, I had no problem standing and getting home, though I was shaken and surprised by the experience. I am grateful that the cane did not choose to self-destruct while I traveled via subway, bus, or air as I often do. As a registered nurse for thirty years, I never heard of this type of accident. I am recovering with the help of a chiropractor, and my back exercises.

I know that canes, as safety devices should not break under the weight of my one hundred and five pounds. Surely, in serving the aging population, you will consider removing this product from the market!

I am interested in your thoughts on this incident.

Sincerely,

Florence Ditlow, R.N.

When the company answered my letter by phone some weeks later, I insinuated to their risk manager that they had made my cane from recycled cola cans. I sent back the defective cane to its maker, who paid for the chiropractic visits that were necessary, due to the fall.

Panchakarma

▼

Scott Gerson, was a passionate proponent of Panchakarma, one component of Ayurvedic medicine, and an ancient Indian method of detoxification. In order to clear toxins from the body, one needs a functional liver. Assuming that the liver is not overburdened by disease, it is capable of converting toxic elements from food, and sources of pollution. Then the kidney will safely excrete these wastes.

Those who devote time to this cleansing practice, do so to rest and renew the body. Rest and relaxation is a key to preventing the body from enduring undue depletion of energy. The mind should rest as well, so practitioners encourage participants to perform Panchakarma in a peaceful, natural setting.

Scott's retreat center was his spacious home in upstate New York, where one could experience a deep rest, which enhanced healing of body, mind, and spirit. Christina, who was a massage therapist, led the therapeutic team. She and Scott were husband and wife. The rooms were minimally furnished, sunny and quiet. In the absence of city stresses and routine, one could explore the woods, and we found time to bask on the sun-drenched patio, while listening to the serenade of warm winds moving through the trees. The large meeting room witnessed early morning Yoga stretching exercise, evening meditation, and after dinner social gatherings. The significance of the many bathrooms became clear when I experienced the treatments, which could best be described as vast oil baths.

I have had many forms of massage, mostly after my illness began. I knew that massage was a circulatory aid, able to facilitate blood flow to the tissues and ease the elimination of toxic wastes. I felt relaxed and strengthened when I had bodywork, but there was much more happening here on an energetic level. One trusted masseuse suggested that from her experience, she knew that memories are capable of being stored. Specifically, she said the body stores memories in the muscle and bone. She had witnessed the emotional release of memory as it *moved out*. Later, I would know how right she was, but this revelation was yet to come.

Massage and adventure were hardly synonymous until I experienced my first Panchakarma treatment. Two therapists worked with me: a man, and a woman. First, I disrobed. *Losing* the laundry was an embarrassing, if necessary ingredient. The absence of all clothing paved the way for cups of sesame massage oil: warm with herbs and truly transforming. I was given nose drops to clear the senses. More sesame oil was scrubbed into my scalp, and then they began the massage. The therapeutic duo stood on opposite sides of the table. At a signal they began making sweeps in unison from my hip to my neck. The first unctuous sweep pressed the air out of my lungs.

"Breathe, Florence, breathe with us," the woman suggested gently. Soon their superficial massage sweeps synchronized their breath to mine. Their long, oiled lunges continued in a path over marma points on the front of my body. Marma points were originally taught to soldiers in ancient India as places where the opponent was vulnerable. Medical sages later utilized the points as targets for massage practitioners to stimulate the body's immune system.

They continued working rapidly. Sweat dripped from the woman's forehead, as the room was hot. Her male counterpart wore a bandana, which was soon soaked. They did not rest until the front of my body and whole scalp was covered with oil. As they were drinking water, a tape of sitar music was turned over in the tape player, and I turned face down. The music lent an ecstatically festive air to this ritual Indian form of touch therapy.

They finished moving through their unique routine in about forty-five minutes. Phase one had left me peaceful, even joyful! The second part involved a body mudpack, which contained specific herbs for my body type. The clay-like material was allowed to dry, and was scraped off. Then the cheery *Panchatechs* proceeded by positioning a steam tent over me, and fastened it to the massage table.

Now my body, warmed by the oil, the friction, and purged of impure matter on the skin's surface, was about to be steamed. The technicians spoke to me freely, since my head was not inside the tent.

I enjoyed the heat, realizing within that hot fog, that I rarely perspire. Toxins, who could say which, food borne, air borne, along with stuck emotion, seemed to dissipate with the beads of cool sweat. My attendant tranquility, and daydreaming were interrupted when the tent was removed twenty minutes later, and I was wrapped in a clean sheet. An oil enema of the variety given with a hand held syringe was prepared to take into the bathroom before leaving the treatment room. It would ease the exit of detoxified waste products, and instill healing herbs. Before the enema, they would attend to my head.

Shirodhara is the name of the next phase of Panchakarma. It is yet more oil, applied to the head by means of a container, which drips it in a stream, onto the forehead. This *third eye* area is thought in Panchakarma practice, to be a key to cognitive clarity; allowing an opening for memories stored from past life wisdom, as well as allowing heightened intuitive thinking.

People at the retreat reported having had visions during Shirodhara. No visions materialized, however, I felt worries somehow drip off my brain. As the last of the warm oil went through my hair, I emerged from the dreamlike state, deeply relaxed, like a ball of *Silly Putty* that pooled on the table, in a state of calm. Each day the ritual treatment was repeated, coaxing the body to let go of what had cluttered it, because the liver, the largest of the body's glands, was cleaning house.

Sharing meals with your oil-washed retreat mates is to be in a rare circle of nurturance. The participants' energy slowly spiraled higher during our stay, with each passing day. The food served at the center was tasty and easily digested. There were few complaints about the fresh fruit, baked veggies, or basmati *kitchadees*, rice combined with legumes and spices, excellent for Panchakarma nourishment, and helpful in the promotion of detoxification. Gallons of filtered water were consumed. Energy and water seemed to be partners.

If anyone grumbled, it was from Scott's advice to stop eating when the stomach was half-full. A partially empty stomach is better able to prepare the food for its digestive fires. Air supports combustion of food and the burning of calories. We were advised to continue to consume soups, vegetable and grain combos for several days following the retreat. This would extend the detoxification. I enjoyed the mildly spiced food, which always included ghee, or clarified butter. I learned to cook with ghee when preparing grain dishes.

Humor probably wasn't a high priority to the Vedic scholars of old, but there it was as I sat in the dining room of that first retreat, in 1996. Scott patiently explained a *special* therapy to me, almost reverent in his delivery of knowledge about the *Shirovasti*. What set me shrieking with laughter was the associated equipment. He would place a large, hard strip of leather around my head; it resembled the headpiece of an Egyptian goddess. After it was secured, it would act as a *bowl*, (my head being the base) for yet more heated, herbal oil.

I couldn't stop laughing. I truly thought he was pulling my leg. Another patient of Scott's, due to receive the special treatment, never blinked as he described how he would prevent oil leakage by packing gauze around the leather, and then duct taping it.

As I was in the throes of a rare laughing jag, I considerately moved to another room so I could laugh while he went on to explain the benefits to my fellow retreat mate.

"Shirovasti is a great thing to do if your problem is in the head. It balances all the doshas. Mental and physical exhaustion, migraines, eye trouble, or anything sensory, even insomnia, can be treated like this. OK. Where did Florence disappear to?"

By now I had regained my composure, "She escaped the ashram!" I yelled into the next room.

The thought of balancing a cylinder of canola oil on my head for half an hour was enough to start more giggles, but we two women with our respective vata problems were successfully treated, with a minimum of oil in the eye. The outcome as one might surmise, was a feeling of calm. Over the years to come, I laughed less and appreciated the entire process as truly meditative.

Panchakarma, is as miraculous as healing can get. The full impact after the four-day course of therapy was reflected in my body. I was fully rested, with extra energy, which somehow compensated for my lack of coordination. Aches and mysterious pains had surfaced along with emotional release. There is no doubt in my mind that the aches I experienced were related to elimination of toxins. We witnessed this in our retreat group and I saw the difference in the sparkle of my formerly tired eyes.

The retreat retrained my skills at meditating, cooking, and sleeping, like Rip Van Winkle. However, I would fail at Yoga. My balance and floor exercises often ended with frustrating, if quiet, tirades. My spiritual teacher, Swami Beyondananda, had dubbed this practice, *Tantrum Yoga*.

Years later, I would discover Bikram Yoga, and succeed. I would be able to do these yoga exercises by holding a ballet bar, and by using a chair. The way was then clear to exercise slowly, stretch, and sweat out toxins.

The time on retreat that I had taken to sit on the grass in the sunny afternoons had restored my connection with the natural world. The earth seemed to say, "I'm changing and you must also be willing to change." The Ayurvedic formula of ancient India is unique in its ability to transform those invested in the desire to be well.

Fancy Channeling

▼

My friend Joan, who had sent me to the Tibetan doctor, Dr. Dhonden, called with another suggestion for healing. She referred me to a hands-on healer who had an office in his Manhattan home.

His name was Manny Cline. He lived in the Lower East side, on the second floor of a house. He was around forty-five, with a tall frame and graying hair. His apartment was very sparsely furnished, without a shred of clutter. I recall three large, calming paintings, with Christian themes, a cross near the treatment table, and the portrait of a power angel in the entryway adorning the walls.

During my appointment, he mentioned having survived a health related ordeal, emerging from that with the discovery that he could heal others. I climbed to the second floor landing, where he ushered me to the living room. After our introductions, he urged me to remove my shoes. He watched me intently, saying a few words that recalled our phone conversation.

"It doesn't matter too much what other doctors have told you about your illness, because I work from a different angle. I think I have an idea about your problem. Is your father alive?" he asked me.

"No, he died a few years ago."

"Well, Florence, your father is here now in spirit. He is concerned about you. His presence is saintly...and he is in a *very* good place."

"He is?" I remarked incredulously, while lying face up on his table. He placed a hand under my back at the heart, while the opposite hand was over my navel. Seated on a folding chair, Manny was uncharacteristically quiet. I felt heat, and a slow electric vibration, which poured long and deeply into my heart.

"You are like a sunken sub, and I'm pouring life into you, but I'm getting that life from God," he added, moving to the foot of the table.

"My father didn't talk to us very conversationally," I slowly said, stunned by his revelations, and the energy, which felt more and more like I was floating. "He was in a lot of pain and I think it distracted and worried him. He spent too much time worrying…" I couldn't continue. I began to cry. I cried and cried.

Minutes later, as I listened through a curtain of grief, I heard Manny say, "You've held part of your father's pain since way back then. It's as though your nervous system is a fabric. It was torn from you, like your father's was torn, and it'll take some time to repair it."

Daddy, a saint, I thought. Mom wouldn't buy it. In fact, I believed all these years that the saint was my mother, and that the only way my father had been able to survive was due to her selfless ministrations. Manny's declarations surfaced as he spent time adding more *life* to my brain, towing the *sub* to the surface.

"Your grief is why the brain is affected. You had a ball of grief in your right foot as well. You will begin to feel the fabric of God in everything."

Manny concluded the ninety-minute laying-on-of-hands session by recommending that I "Go to what feels warm."

Mexico fit Manny's description of warm to a tee. I longed for a hot and humid vacation with Honey. I am lying on the yellow, surf-milled sand, staring out at the turquoise ocean in the distance. I had a vision of my father, the week before he died in 1992. He was dancing, dancing, ballet-like, in a gossamer cape. I was dazed then, not by the proximity of his death, but by the possibility of his dance routine. Never had I seen my father dance!

I ponder the father-daughter connection. I think back to the breath work session at the nurses' convention, when Daddy *was present* in the room and the therapist, suggested I say to Daddy that I was OK, that I was safe. My father worried about me? And he was worrying from a *very good place*? When he was in this world, he did not seem to be all that concerned about me. I went through a divorce when I lived far from home. This motivated him to write a several letters, which expressed concern. The letter was an invitation to come home, that the door was open, if I needed a place to go.

I thought of Maria's instruction, when she told me about a *place inside that was never nurtured*. A place never nurtured. I remembered fleeting jealousy of my friends who had actual conversations with their fathers, instead of being given countless work directives. I remembered Daddy, speaking politely to his co-workers, but not often to his own family. Being a reliable breadwinner was enough. He worked a twelve-hour day, came home for dinner, and then went to bed. I often awakened to the sound of his truck exiting the drive at 4 A.M., out into the gray dawn.

I think about my saintly mother, who would never claim sainthood, who had to try to communicate to Daddy across the chasm of his pain. Now, a man who refers to himself as a *fancy channel* says that my father has a saintly presence. The breeze is salty, and a seabird lands near my lounge chair by the vacant pool.

"I'm going to go back to Manny," I told the seabird, who looked right at me, as if interested. The yellow-pink sunsets were wraparound, unlike the views from our New York apartment.

Honey and I returned sun soaked from our vacation. One of the first things I did was to make an appointment for energy work. If Manny was compassionate the first time, now he was a comedian. Everything he said made me laugh.

"Humor is a basic requirement. They don't let you into heaven without it," he told me. "The heart is what matters, not the facade most people buy into. You know, people act just like they've been brainwashed."

Even when he worked on me, the comedy didn't stop. He started as before, running *life* into my heart, then moving his folding chair around the treatment table, going wherever I needed to have the previously identified cold spots, removed. He placed his hands on my feet, and that familiar heat seemed to go up my spine.

"I'm glad you quit working," he said. "You wouldn't believe my patients who've been drained by CEOs! I see the problem in the brain, Florence." Now he was sitting at the head of the table, so he could place his hands on my forehead, and on the back of my head. I imagined myself to be healing my cerebellum. That is the portion of the brain that deals with balancing the body.

"It's as though interlocking parts of the brain are disconnected. What I do here helps it to congeal properly. You will live. The body knows how to heal. You can do this. What you're doing is cleaning up your father's work addiction."

Next he moved his chair to work on my legs. "The human body amazes me. Compare it to medical science's knowledge of it. Now, medical science is like a lean-to. The body is like the Space Shuttle. So much smarter."

And then a new observation from Manny, as I was about to get down from the treatment table, something only surprising, because Manny had never met my husband.

"Your husband's love for you is genuine. It almost makes me cry. I suggest that you fall in love with him all over again."

That session was not energizing. Walking home felt as if I'd strapped a brick to each shoe. I was not feverish, but his clearing of the cold had left me feeling very warm on a cool spring day. Wending my halting, cane-supported way back home, via subway, I was thinking about Manny's opinion of medical science. I remembered what he had said about my father. Inside my apartment, I sat down to sip my cup of hot *Ayurvedic* tea, and wondered how I could help to honor, and to heal myself.

My father had visited me at least twice, stopping his heavenly dance, and entering the sessions I had created in order to heal myself. Was it possible that he was trying to get my attention? To say, "Keep your focus but don't over-do it, like I did."

As the chamomile steam rose against my face, I entered a contemplative stillness, where I was wishing for some way, thinking, but not too much…

Out of my mouth came a whispered, "I love you, Daddy." I silently went to the bookshelf, miraculously locating a videotape compiled by my brother, Jim. I pulled it off a top shelf with my cane. On it were a series of home movies, taken by my father. When Daddy died, Jim gave a copy to each of our family members.

I thought that if I could view these movies through my father's eyes, I might come closer to knowing the man. Using the mindset of someone I had met who had studied neurolinguistic programming, I decided for a time, to *become* my father! I inserted the cassette into the VCR, and pushed *play*. There they were.

The birthday parties. The sandbox. Our dog, Queenie. Through the camera's lens, he looked at me in the playpen.

My father, in a rare shot taken by my mother, pulls the rope on our sled, and *runs* as my sister and I scream in this silent black and whiteness of a winter landscape.

I see surely, he photographs with love. Perhaps it's a normal father's loving pride that urges this type of photo session. Perhaps not. I was a very fortunate child. Fortunate to be held, fortunate to be taken on the early tricycle outings in front of the bakery. Fortunate to have known those he caught lovingly on film: the love of my great-grandparents, grandparents, aunts, uncles, a sister, two brothers and of course, Mom.

He photographs with love.

The images continue to flash across the screen. It's the fifties in Technicolor. My baby brother, wearing a floor-length pink dress, parades in front of my great-grandmother, who's sitting outside our house, hair in a bun, neatly dressed, and clutching a small panda. My sister holds my oldest brother, Chris, who is nearly as big as she. Beside her, I hold a treasured doll that is losing its hair.

Without warning, I am crying. Crying from the depths of my soul. Crying in different ways for different reasons. First, there were tears of gratitude for this family of mine.

Next I am grieving for the loss of the man who had been my *first* father: the guy who was so happy to have me as his daughter, the one who shared in the fun that was the substance of my childhood. The one I sat next to on the couch to watch these home movies when they were brand new. The one who let me help him dig the garden, where we uncovered a nest of bunnies. Four years ago, I had grieved for the seventy-two-year-old *second* father, but now perhaps, I was observing the *third* man, the spirit which had become *saintly*.

The deranged man, the man who did not express emotion well, the man I had stopped communicating with when I was eleven, the man who had dropped out of my world, unless I spoke of work. That man was born from pain. My mother took care of this man in almost constant pain, for most of their married life, only relenting when his demands began to compromise her own health.

"I know why you're doing this!" he screamed, that day my seventy-two-year-old mother put him in a nursing home. "You've got another man! You dump me so's ya can run off with another man!"

In all of the health-challenged pain of his later years, I had forgotten about the *first* father, the one who had a heart that was not yet sucked dry by suffering. My memories washed out of the video like clues written in indelible ink, now coming into focus. Predictably, the memories of my father were linked to work. He needed to work as a livelihood and a therapy.

The Have a Heart Trap was a device probably invented by some humane society, so that rats could be caught, and then set free.

Daddy's direction to my brothers: "You boys take this Have a Heart trap. There's a mouse inside. Hold it against the exhaust pipe of my truck. Ha! Ha! He'll never know what hit'm."

That was how he had disposed of mice, daring enough to venture into his antique business of his later years. When he *retired* in the 1970's, he started dealing in antiques. He could be actively involved in work, although the crippling effect of arthritis barely permitted him the strength to lift a phone receiver. Unfortunately, this work also required the help of my mother and brothers. They stoked the wood burning stove, lifted Victorian furniture wardrobes, visited customers' murky basements, and performed the dreaded arrangement of dusty paintings or stuffed great horned owls.

Nothing, certainly not health, was more important than work. Around the clock work, which distracted my father from pain, served as physical therapy for multiple arthritic joints, and psychotherapy for a one-track mind.

The videotape came to an abrupt end. But something within me had only begun. The home movie archive had unlocked long-forgotten memories, which had released the powerful tears of healing.

That evening, I reminisced with Genady, who had met my father a short time before he died. I told him about the feeling after the energy session and how the leaden feeling of my feet was just now clearing out. I described my *first* father's ability to be involved with us. He was once playful; it's there on film! He'd been there to teach me to ride a two-wheeler at seven, and he taught me to do my multiplication tables. Being with him used to be a pleasure. Days later, after the heat of my treatment dissipated, I continued reflecting on that night at the movies. I began loving my father, the saintly one, the one free of pain in death, as I had never been able to do in his workaholic years when our tasks divided us.

In the midst of this reinterpretation of my relationship with Daddy, I did indeed fall in love with Honey, all over again.

Energy

▼

"Everything is energy."

Rosalyn Bruyere

Energy! It's a simple concept, simple to feel, to know what it's like, yet difficult to describe the cellular mechanisms scientifically.

I recall the simple structural make-up of our cells. Looking at one cell reveals the mission-control portion, or nucleus, which tells component parts what to do. Surrounding the nucleus, the cytoplasm, contains numerous tiny cellular workers ready to carry out the mission. The energy worker is the mitochondria. These are fluid filled bodies, able to change their shapes as desired. Enzymes connected to mitochondria are responsible for converting glucose and other molecules into energy.

Simply stated, that apple you ate had some simple sugar in it that became energy, thanks in part, to the powerhouse called mitochondria.

I know what energy feels like. I was bursting with energy as a child, running, biking, and yes, laughing. Later, I took up jogging, and stayed with it for ten years. Jogging gave me an aerobic education in oxygenation. It reminded me that breathing provides the body with high levels of oxygen, thus infusing all of the cells with energy, which is one of the benefits of exercise.

Now, Manny, my fancy channel, had also given me an energy infusion, one that was restful, rather than stimulating, calming, rather than stirring. This sensation was similar to the acupuncture treatments, when I enjoyed a deep rest, the deepest rest I had ever experienced without sleep. T'ai chi also infuses me with restful energy, and at the same time it helps to stabilize my balance and keep me grounded.

The slow calm motion of hand, and then foot, also improved my coordination. What's more, flowing chi is good for the immune system, as is the setting on the East River, where our group met. Here we could listen to the boat-churned waves, slapping against the sea wall, as well as experience the increased energy that a group provides.

In the spring of 1995, I wanted to create more of this restful energy that I had received from Manny, acupuncture, and T'ai chi. I had been marinating much too long in the stress of the big city. During my years in the allopathic medical world, I had come to rely on the American Holistic Nurses Association as an oasis in the desert of the hard-driving health care system of the nineties— a system that was capable of causing *dis-ease* in the very people who had entered the profession to help cure it.

My feelings were born out of the frustration of working in hospitals where too many tasks were assigned to too few healthcare workers, and where the standard medical model was largely outmoded. The nurse who works in the hospital environment is like a concert conductor, orchestrating the dispensing of healthcare to the separate rooms inhabited by the patients. She must conduct a multitude of tasks accurately, in a timely fashion.

My caring activities as a registered nurse have included observing debilitated surgical patients, administering complex medications, presiding over monitoring devices, keeping meticulous records, and educating patients in their own self-care. This rarely left any time for teaching patients how to avoid illness, and future trips to the hospital. In my opinion, the patient who returned to the hospital soon after discharge was a sign that the hospital had failed to educate them in self-care.

Hospitals sometimes claimed to value prevention of illness, but their actions communicated otherwise. They were promoting practices reimbursed by insurance companies, such as testing, surgery, and diagnostic procedures. Reimbursement is more difficult to get for preventative measures, which administrators usually resist making available. Today, more practitioners of every persuasion, as well as more healthcare institutions and hospitals have allied themselves with holistic healing practices.

As a holistic nurse, I believe that true health takes into consideration the body, the mind, and the spirit. We as healthcare practitioners must be very conscious of our own needs. Interestingly enough, as I became more conscientious in my beliefs, I realized that a cultural shift in healthcare was happening concurrently in the minds of a lot of other people. Friends who had never heard of Panchakarma, or Ayurvedic practices, had heard of detoxification. People no longer turned up their noses at the notion of holistic healers. There was less sniggering at the mention of esoteric practices, even if one didn't understand the mechanism that made the practice *work*.

Health food stores began to serve growing numbers of customers at the supplement shelf, and I watched them pour into the juice bar. We holistic nurses were no longer a lonely voice in an allopathic medical world. The public had joined us and brought their money with them.

I lacked the required energy to travel to the summer 1996 American Holistic Nurses convention, so instead I took a three-day course called Healing Touch, in nearby Madison, Connecticut. Healing Touch originated when Janet Mentgen, an R.N., became interested in the work of various healers she had met and studied with. Eventually, using earlier energy-healing techniques as an inspiration, she built her own system of bioenergetic healing.

She started training others to do these healing techniques, and set up a network of trainers throughout the world, so that anyone interested in this healing process could learn it. A Healing Touch certificate program was offered through the American Holistic Nurses Association.

The nurse who conducted my introductory course was from Canada, and spent much of her time training others in the techniques. Alexandra Johnson began by teaching us some of the theories of quantum physics. In a nutshell, each part of the body relates to every other part. Furthermore, the body relates directly to the environment when it consumes air and food. It follows, that parts of Earth relate to the whole planet, and that the Earth in turn, relates to the cosmos. In essence, everything is interdependent upon everything else. In sum: all is one.

She then showed our class of twenty-five students, how to assess energy needs, and how to replenish energy. She demonstrated exercises that alleviate trauma and pain. The human hand is the key to Healing Touch, and most discussion focused on the use of the hand as a tool of energy. We learned to sense irregularities in the energy field with the use of our hands. These irregularities could act as traps for bioelectric energy, draining to the general health. A headache could send out hot waves that were easily felt by my hand. When the person receiving the treatment, intended, for instance, to release the headache pain, simple placement or movement of my hands on the head was capable of doing just that.

I felt this already in the Panchakarma detoxification, and in Manny's art of moving *life* force. But Healing Touch was distinguished by a few differences. The client was involved more so in establishing a focus or intention. Here the mind begins to set up the subconscious for a desirable future outcome. The practitioner learns to become connected to the earth or *grounded*, which facilitates the movement of energy. Rubbing one's palms together is one way to get grounded. Perhaps the biggest surprise was the number of ways available to move this bioelectric energy, without touching the client's body.

Our first practice session found me playing the role of a client lying on the treatment table, while my partner cleared my energy field. After a short focus for grounding the practitioner, she began to move her hands slowly, about twelve inches above my body. She repeatedly passed her hands from my head to my foot, palms facing me; her hands could feel my energy field change after about twenty passes. Relaxing into a mental vacation, I enjoyed losing track of time. The effect of grounding helped to stabilize my balance. My partner offered me a cup of water, pulling me back into reality, and soon I was playing the practitioner role.

I sensed a stagnant area around her navel. Within a few minutes of moving my hands through the energy field, I could no longer feel that *break* in the continuity of her energy field. As one of the students observed, it felt like the energy field had become *smooth as glass*. As the instructor proceeded with other techniques, I realized that the power of touch, and the intention to ease discomfort that Alexandra advocated, was what I had practiced all those years that I stood at the bedside of anxious hospitalized patients. Knowing that holding someone's hand could ease pain, or speed the effect of pain medication; I held a patient's hand while she was attached to a cardiac monitor. With calming touch, her previously erratic heart rhythm normalized.

Now, in Healing Touch (HT), I saw that by placing my hands above my partner's body at her energy centers, her human bioelectric field, or aura, was affected. I did not need a machine to provide proof of the benefit; my proof was in her smile, in her sparkling eyes, and even in her hair, which had a new shine.

A uniquely intriguing key to the class participants' interest in HT was the study of the energy centers. Known as Chakras, there is a center of energy approximating the location of all major organ systems. According to HT, each center corresponds to a color in the spectrum of light. We focused on the appropriate colors for a self-healing technique, and practiced while sitting in a chair. Beginning as usual, by grounding ourselves, we then placed our own hands on the largest energy centers. We followed our instructor as she first placed her hands on her ankle and knee, focusing on the color red. In about thirty seconds, I began feeling a pulsing sensation in both hands, which cued me to move to a higher point. We repeated this process, moving up the body, finally placing our palms on our forehead, and on the crown of the head.

"Orange, your hands are at the navel. Yellow, your hands are over the solar plexus, or spleen area. Green, the heart. Sky-blue, the throat. Dark indigo-blue, the forehead. White, is the top of the head," Alexandra guided.

The color reflected the various frequencies of light. At times I have been drawn to certain colors, predominantly red. Red happens to correspond to the legs, and therefore to grounding and to survival. It comes as no surprise that wearing red appears to help me stay balanced, both emotionally and physically.

Besides practicing all of the techniques of HT on others in the class, I received treatment in return. This was important, our instructor said, not only for self-care, but to enable the practitioner to feel the effect of the work. I was given quite a souvenir, too. There was an offer from a manufacturer of therapeutic tables, for participants to purchase such a table at a substantial price reduction.

As I considered the possible uses of that bright purple table, my mouth seemed to move robot-like, as if freed from its connection to my brain. It mumbled in a monotone, "Do you take plastic money?" and I came to my senses as I signed the credit slip. Somehow, I was intended to have that simple tool of energy work. Little did I know, that before a month went by, five people, myself included, would receive an HT treatment on the purple table.

One technique that would become a regular component of my healing repertoire was lymphatic drainage. More than any other self-applied technique, I relied on this exercise to clear toxins from the lymph circulation. It works by moving the hands in the air, above the body, first, down from the shoulder, legs, and then up from the neck. In so doing, one may activate lymphatic circulation, as if you had stretched a rubber band, until it snapped.

I was a ball of energy when I got off the homeward bound Amtrak train, three days later. It wasn't long before situations presented themselves to prove the efficacy of Healing Touch.

My first out-of-class, hands-on-healing session took place on an interstate highway. My first patient was Honey. My husband is allergic to pollen, big time. In through the open car window came a Tsunami of a pollen problem. His left eye began itching, and then swelled up like a Puff Adder.

"Let's stop!" he said, looking at the affected eye in the rear view mirror. He was clearly in pain.

"Let's keep going," I urged, "I just saw an *H* sign that a hospital is a mile away."

We checked into the quiet emergency room, where the receptionist told us to sit in the waiting area. We found a secluded corner to sit down, and I began to treat Genady's eye with my newly acquired techniques.

This called for a *laser* technique, which I applied with my index finger, directing the energy into the tear duct, intending to help drain the swelling. Minutes passed, and my *laser* finger began to move rhythmically, almost independently of me, and easily around the eye. Five minutes later I sensed that something was changing. Genady's posture relaxed as I began working on the head, and then on the whole body, as practiced in the Healing Touch class.

I stood in front of his chair directing the energy. I was feeling an intense heat releasing from the affected eye. I asked him to breathe deeply. The pain had diminished. I proceeded to work again, directing energy from my palm, over his closed, swollen, red eye. With the opposite hand, I worked with the energy center at the forehead, calming the sense of sight.

Fifteen minutes had passed, and I noticed that the people at the admission desk were craning their necks, and watching me furtively, probably rolling their own eyes at this *goofy family member*. I tried not to think how my antics must look to them, but concentrated instead on sweeping the irritation out.

"Which eye is it?" asked the doctor, when we were in the exam room. He moved in for a close look.

Healing Touch, applied to the amazing machinery of the human body, changed the appearance of Genady's formerly frog-like eye, to normal, in less than forty-five minutes. Each time I applied the techniques, either to myself or to others, I became more convinced of the value of energy work.

There is a web of energy around the body that is an integral part of the body. I can describe it as egg shaped, unseen, and yet as important as the egg is to a baby chick. Treating this field of energy with the help of a practitioner, or as self-practice, has great potential for healing body and mind.

Realistically, I couldn't get frequent HT treatments, but I could do daily T'ai chi. Ancient energy practices such as T'ai chi were the basis for HT, and contributed much to my powerful prescription for healing. The rewards were my flexibility, calmness, and a sense of integrity.

I did T'ai chi at the homeless center, as a way to center myself prior to the weekly laugh sessions. Often, as participants drifted in, they silently joined in, shadowing my slowly moving body. This was a good beginning for group interaction. Warmer months permitted me to do my routine outside, often barefooted, as I plugged my energy field into the Roosevelt Island earth. My body weaves slightly as I begin, but after the opening exercises, I feel steadier. Sometimes passing children stare at me, but I just smile, or if they are very young, I make a funny face. The energy practices calm my mind, help with my balance, and tone my nervous system.

I decided that energy work was important enough to practice it every day. My interest prompted me to take several additional Healing Touch courses, which expanded my knowledge of energy work, preparing me to heal others. Years later I would have the privilege of further energy study with Rev. Rosalyn Bruyere, a master of hands-on healing. As I recalled Maria's early advice, honoring myself was to be a key to healing. Energy studies and practices certainly have assisted me in the quest for wellness. It is a field that I had only minimal knowledge of as a nurse, when I was free of illness.

Dental Metals: The Missing Link

▼

The winter of 1996 found me following the suggestion of Dr. Gerson: to hibernate. I avoided the icy streets of my neighborhood, emerging only for an occasional appointment. This time I met with Sandra Senzon, a dental hygienist, in private practice. Sandy had been treating me ever since I stepped into her office for cleaning, years before.

Sandy had a unique gift: she put humor and healing into dental hygiene.

"People eat wrong then stress out! Whadaya get? Decay. It never fails."

In her spare time she dressed as the tooth fairy for children's dental education programs. She was the perfect practitioner for my gum problem. In 1995 she saw that my gums were inflamed and had receded below the crowns, which had been fitted in 1991.

"Florence," she said, gesturing with her violet latex gloved hand, "Your problem is only with the teeth that are crowned. Maybe we can have them replaced."

After several futile attempts to treat the gingivitis, which included scraping the pockets of gum tissue, she suggested that I look into replacing the crowns. I found a dentist who wanted me to have a look at some videos that addressed replacement of crowns, and metal-related gingivitis. He used these patient information videos to substantiate his position regarding dental amalgam revision.

Genady accompanied me to see the dentist who we will refer to as Dr. Paynow. The sidewalk was a sheet of ice as I skidded into the dentist's office. In the waiting room, we viewed four videos, each of which were based on studies that illustrated the horrors of mercury.

The announcer said that while mercury has long been a staple of dentistry and has preserved many millions of teeth, it has the ability to get into body tissues through vaporization, inhaling and swallowing saliva.

We saw a sheep with mercury amalgam in its teeth (probably the sheep ate too much refined sugar) and x-rays, which showed that the metal had apparently migrated from the teeth to the liver.

Gingivitis is only one of the signs of heavy metal toxicity. Patients on the videotapes complained of transitory fatigue, anxiety, and chronic fatigue syndrome. There was a presentation by Dr. Hal Huggins, the dentist credited with establishing a connection between heavy metals in dentistry and autoimmune diseases. He set up a center in Colorado in the 1980's to help people with that set of problems. He has taught dentists and others his protocols for the removal of dental metals.

One man went to the Huggins Center in a wheelchair and had the amalgam fillings removed. He was filmed at a later date, walking, now independent of his mobility device. A woman with multiple sclerosis had her dental amalgams removed, also hoping to get relief from her symptoms, but she felt no improvement. It seems that Dr. Huggins has seen people with weak immunity such as rheumatoid arthritis, cardiovascular complaints, birth defects, and a host of miscellaneous digestive and psychological difficulties improve when amalgams are removed.

A partial list of symptoms shown in the videos as being linked to mercury accumulation in the tissues included: numbness and tingling in fingers and toes, hand tremors, uncoordinated muscular movements, memory loss and mood disturbances. Dr. Huggins attributed the clearing of vague headache, sinus, and gastrointestinal complaints, among other symptoms, to the removal of amalgams containing mercury.

Mercury was said to disrupt chromosomes in the white blood cells, making cell reproduction impaired. Since white cells are instrumental in defending the body against invaders, the immune system suffers.

However, the announcer on the video also cautioned us that doing a dental restoration was no guarantee of the alleviation of symptoms.

We looked up as Dr. Paynow emerged from his office, after Genady and I had watched this dental film festival. He looked at my mouth, noting the amalgams.

"It's no wonder that you are sick. If I were you, I'd come back, at least for x-rays."

I closed my mouth, and replied, "Let's just say I remove my crowns…they seem to be the real problem. I didn't have any symptoms until the crowns were fitted."

"Well, I'll tell you the way I work. I do the entire mouth. I believe in removing *all* of the metal," he stated with authority.

"Can you give an estimate of what that would cost?" I asked. I supposed that by redoing the crowns, I'd at least get a cure of the gum disease.

"I'd say it would cost about the same as a new car."

I wondered aloud, "What do new cars cost? I'm driving a Volkswagen with a hundred thousand miles on it."

"Oh, about $20,000. When can you come in for x-rays?"

Gulp. My husband didn't like Dr. Paynow, even before the cost estimate; he thought the man did little to evoke trust. I was most struck by the dramatic demonstration that implied that there was a link between certain neurological symptoms and amalgam use in dentistry.

My former dentist had moved to another city. I now recalled that my last visit to him in 1991, to have the offending crowns fitted, was followed by the insidious onset of symptoms, two months later. The *mouth* was where my symptoms began, with eventually so much saliva I had to swallow just to finish a sentence. Gum problems followed. I remembered the tests performed by the neurologist, showing heavy metals to be *within normal limits*, but now I felt certain that the metal was responsible for my problem. The symptoms surreptitiously began soon after the dental metal exposure. I felt I hadn't struck gold, but it felt great. What I'd hit on was mercury.

ALS or Primary lateral sclerosis, I thought, is a name for a set of symptoms. The cause could arise from hereditary tendencies, but suppose *acquired* neurological disorders could be traced to mercury and other heavy metals?

The week following my visit to Dr. Paynow, I began phoning people who had had their mercury amalgam removed. One was a fellow chiropractic patient, one a satisfied *Paynow* patient, and one was an employee of the Huggins center, but none of these had neurological difficulties; their situations were not as precarious as mine. The herbalist I had come to know, admonished, "Don't take chances. You might make things worse."

I got a similar message when I spoke with a dentist at the Huggins center by phone. He explained that a specific protocol must be followed for replacing mercury amalgams with non-toxic materials, otherwise the things really might get worse.

I needed more data to be able to make an educated decision. In the meantime, I would continue with the Ayurvedic detoxification as well as with my exercise. Finally, I reached a point of overwhelming confusion on the dental issue and decided against making a decision for the time being. But rejoice! I had outlived my credit card.

1997

My 1997 prescription included:
  T'ai chi: 3-4 times weekly
  Energy work
  Ayurvedic routines
  Tibetan herbs
  Fifteen-minute meditations: twice daily
  Juicing and Vegan diet
  Waterobics weekly
  Humor

Dream...
Macy's Celebration
I enter Macy's and observe the following scene:
Gilda Radner, in her Roseanne Rosanadana, personality of *Saturday Night Live*, calls out to the cashiers.
"Your next transaction will be (she inhales deeply) a new high, a pinnacle, a landmark."

I go to a cashier although I haven't bought anything. The cashier is excited.

Gilda continues, "When your cash register opens, no price will appear. Instead, you will see the words: MACY'S...MACY'S...MACY'S." As if that was their cue, about a dozen cashiers on the main floor rang up registers in unison. The registers looked new, but had those *ca ching*, chinging bells of the pre-computer age. The dreamscape shifts. Now I am the guest of honor at a Macy's boardroom table, with twenty employees.

"The big man's comin' in," whispers the employee to my right.

The big man turns out to be Zippy the Pinhead, who is a cartoon character by Bill Griffith. Zippy, a favorite of mine, is a bald, pinheaded man, who has a habit of wearing a yellow, polka dotted dress. He is known for his enjoyment of glazed donuts, and meditation before the dryers in laundromats.

Now, Zippy gives me *exciting* news.

I emerge from sleep. But the dream had not announced the news, and I hadn't been in Macy's since I bought a straw hat for the honeymoon in 1994.

Interpretation: I will be making a sizable purchase.

The WBAI radio station was my lunch accompaniment. As I chewed kale, and rice, that is, blackened kale I had sautéed in garlic and ginger, I heard the voice of dentist Dr. Hal Huggins, the major proponent for amalgam removal in America. This was the Dr. Huggins of the dental videos. Gary Null, a New York health activist, was interviewing him. I listened avidly to his message, which warned against root canal procedures. He said research showed that the portion of the tooth that remains following this procedure is a potentially toxic area, capable of harboring anaerobic bacteria. No one needs anaerobic bugs. I had one root canal, done in 1991. Later in the interview, he briefly mentioned studies linking neuromuscular diseases to the presence of amalgams in our teeth.

Dr. Huggins had actually been able to measure mercury vapor from patients' amalgam fillings by using a Bacharach mercury detector. Patients had exhibited amalgam tattoos or staining of the gum adjacent to an amalgam-filled tooth. The dentist reminded listeners that people with strong immune systems could endure the exposure to these metals perhaps with no symptoms. Dr. Huggins mentioned the chronic illnesses I had previously seen on the dental videos.

terone decline after menopause. I was already taking estrogen and Dr. Levin recommended I add progesterone, which may be applied as a cream.

Chelation:

Chelation means *to claw out*. I was given a trial of DMPS chelation, to check for tolerance, DMPS being an abbreviation for the substance: 2-3-dimercapto-1-propane sulfonic acid. This intravenous, IV, procedure lasted about two hours, leaving me feeling more energetic than when it began. The following day I was really dragging my feet, presumably because the chelation also takes nutrients along with the metal. The procedure includes a second infusion of nutrients on the day after the DMPS IV, in order to replace those essential nutrients lost in the act of flushing out the heavy metals.

When I received the test results, I learned that I had high levels of metal in my tissues. There was so much mercury that the reading went *off the scale*.

Dr. Levin explained that metal tends to gravitate to body fat near nerve tissue. Problems arise when it blocks normal nerve transmission. Metal in the liver obstructs the detoxification of environmental pollutants, which normally would be excreted. This realization partially explained my gastrointestinal symptoms and fatigue.

Ironically, this was good news! It pointed to the source of my problem, as well as gave me a hopeful intervention, one that would be helpful, even to someone diagnosed with Primary Lateral Sclerosis.

Removing my dental metals was indicated, and now, I was thrilled to go to the dentist. I could hardly wait! But my eagerness for x-rays, drilling, and yes, extraction, would bow to discernment. Alas, learning to wait had seemed to be a veiled lesson. I had listened to the radio, the Huggins video, and to the wisdom of Dr. Levy, an M.D., associated with the Huggins center. The message was: if you are sick from heavy metals, educate yourself about detoxification and then proceed slowly.

The Huggins Center in Colorado, gave me three dentists' phone numbers, and all three had been trained there. I was happy with my first choice, Terry Bellman. He was experienced in the area of metal toxicity in dentistry, used only materials compatible with my body chemistry, and worked near my neighborhood. Ironically, thanks to Dr. Bellman's competent counseling, I chose to remove all of my old fillings, as well as the crowns. In so doing, I followed the Huggins's formula, and paid less than half of the cost estimated by Dr. Paynow.

It has been said that the environment in which one is treated may be another form of therapy. I am sure that this is true. I was privileged to have calm, and caring environments all along my path. For this I thank the office staffs, as well as the practitioners.

I was to space the dental visits so that my immune system would not be unnecessarily overloaded, by learning to use my *Circaseptuan rhythm*. This meant avoiding making appointments with seven, fourteen, twenty-one days between them, because according to the Circaseptuan rhythm, these are the days when the immune system is at its weakest following the major stress of the dental revision. Instead, I was instructed by Dr. Bellman to do a follow-up appointment fifteen days after the previous one. Therefore, if I went to my first visit on a Monday, the second visit was to follow fifteen days later, on a Tuesday.

My dental visits were synchronized with my doctor visits in the following way. I would arrive at the doctor's office, where my vital signs would be checked. Then an intramuscular injection of the chelating agent, DMPS, was administered. The DMPS was insurance against mercury getting into my system during the amalgam removal procedure.

DMPS pulls metal out of the tissues into the bloodstream, then it is excreted in the urine. Dr. Levin said metals are also excreted in the stool, and sweat. Every time DMPS is taken, one needs to measure the outgoing metals with each treatment. So, a twenty-four hour urine collection was in order. Every patient was handed an orange box with a handle, as well they were reminded, "Save all urine!" I then got into a cab and took a one-mile ride to my dental visit, where the metal on one tooth would be removed. This tooth then received a non-toxic filling.

I backpacked the urine collection to the office, the next morning on the subway. On quiet days when people were half-asleep in their seats, I could hear urine audibly sloshing around on my back, with every lurch of the train.

Making my way through the doctor's office with the cane, I took a seat, and noticed that entertaining reading matter was available, in the form of a handout. There was a list of substances found to contain mercury. Taken from Huggins's book, with the catchy title, *It's All In Your Head,* the handout described mercury as the single most toxic metal ever investigated. Among the common sources of mercury to beware of exposure, the list read:

Large saltwater fish and shellfish
Some waterproof mascara
Some hair dyes
Some Calamine Lotion
Mercurochrome
Some nasal sprays
Lead mercury solder
Many paints with mercuric oxide
Ethyl mercury chloride wood preservatives
Some photographic solutions
Some tile cement
Some fungicides, herbicides, and insecticides

I put down the sheet of paper, making a mental note to read the label on my hair coloring.

"I have no mercury in my teeth," said the man to my right, who looked about sixty, as he pointed to his front teeth. "I was tested for it. My problem was that I like to eat fish: cod, tuna, and shellfish. I was contaminated with mercury though, because the fish swam in it."

I was sitting next to him in Dr. Levin's clinic infusion room. Our IVs dripped in unison.

"Did you have your teeth measured for electricity? Mine measured zero!" he beamed, over his New York Times.

I answered, "Yeah, I had measurements done…my worst was a minus sixty-four."

What he meant was that teeth repaired with metals usually generate an electrical current, which may be measured by an ammeter. I knew this from reading Huggins's aforementioned book.

Huggins wrote about the current produced by a tooth containing a filling of amalgam metals in contact with saliva, and how dentists should use readings of these currents to define the best order for amalgam replacement. According to him, the most dangerous amalgams, those with the highest readings, in people like me, should be removed first and replaced with a benign filling. I would begin work on the tooth holding the highest negative charge, (-64) and then we would work down to the next highest negative reading. Huggins's experience indicated that those who had the most severe illness also tended to have high negative amalgam currents.

We compared dental adventures among the small array of folks, sitting close together in the small infusion room, our only similarity, the ever-present orange jugs at our feet. A few office patients were undergoing dental revisions and chelation, as I was. One woman commuted by train from Boston, staying in town for the two-day treatment. She was sure that chelation had helped her to survive cancer. She believed that her immune system was under attack due to the amount of metal in her mouth and body.

She said, gesturing with her free arm, "Funny how mercury is dangerous enough to be brought in, in a steel case, brought out of the office in a biohazard box, but they can put it inside your mouth!"

Most of my IV companions, however, were too tired to talk, or too distracted.

Genady usually walked me to the doctor's office, because of my unpredictable balance and lack of energy, which placed me in the walking shadow category. Now safe from the erratic nature of commuters and the train, Genady left me at the door where I was met by a very helpful doorman, who assisted me to the elevator with lots of humor.

"Makin' another delivery?" he would say with a Brooklyn accent, gesturing at my sloshing container.

I bet that man has witnessed thousands of these jugs going in and out of here, I sighed, as the lift brought me to the seventh floor. This refreshing kindness happened to me regularly in this big city, full of humor, yet often thought of as indifferent.

One time, creeping along from the doctor's Fifty-Seventh Street office, I reached the curb, to flag down a cab. Before I could raise my arm, a large man leaped out, hailing a yellow cab and then opening the door for me. A familiar smile lit his eyes.

"Don't I know you?" I asked, combing my brain for where we might have met.

"I'm Mike Sharp…you've seen me in movies…and I'm always a bad guy there. In reality, I'm good. See?" he said, gesturing for me to enter my cab. It was the first time I ever met a movie star.

Fortified by Genady's assistance and New York's uncharacteristic gestures of goodwill, I created as pleasant a stay at the doctor's office as possible. Once hooked to the IV for chelation, I began visualizing my goal. I imagined two *helpers*, twin workmen in denim overalls, with a sign reading: Men at Work. Each held an iridescent hoop, which they drew down over my body. Synchronized with my breath, their hoops pulled out all the metal, easily and effortlessly.

I mentally blocked out the very abrasive man to my left who made business calls while his IV was infusing. I found myself visualizing his cell phone disconnected, and after ten minutes, disconnected and no longer in service! I ignored the frail Chinese man who snored across the room, swallowed up in his cocoon of a sweater.

When on the following day, I received the solution that would replace the nutrients, I asked the *Men at Work* to get working, to use their hoops to replace the nutrients, which had been extracted by the chelation. On the advice of both the Huggins Center, and Dr. Levin, who both believed it helped fortify the immune system, and speeded healing, I tried intravenous Vitamin C. I felt just the same with or without the dozen C drips.

After four months of medical/dental drill, and the removal of five offending crowns and four amalgams circa the fifties, I felt a small surge of energy. I was a lighter, brighter me.

Nothing was instantaneous. Everything had been incremental but I was sure that something had clicked, because a major shift had resulted: gone was the anxiety, which had seized me every time I had gone out alone. Whether this anxiety was based on the experience I had with the gentleman knocking me over, or the ability of the wind to throw me off balance, I didn't care. The fear had been extracted, disappearing with the amalgam removal.

The question that is often posed to me is, "Did you sue the dentist who did the toxic crowns?"

Discovering the cause of my illness, and needing to have funds to perform the dental/medical detoxification, I gave it careful consideration. Fatigue had made a great impact, and energy was in short supply. The dentist in question had moved out of the area. I had to choose the priority of saving my health, and I put all of my effort toward that. One year into the process, I questioned several lawyers about the problem. They answered that they would be willing to take the case, but unequivocally felt that the chances of winning were slim.

Instead of suing, I did something different. First I located the dentist. I decided to inform him of the harm he had unknowingly inflicted. I wrote him a letter describing the state of my health, which had demanded that I divest myself of his toxic root canal and crowns. I enclosed the itemized bill from Dr. Bellman. This letter was businesslike rather than threatening. It requested that he help to defray my mounting medical costs.

The office replied, "We have no record of having you as a patient." I sent proof in the form of detailed facts about my case. I also had the x-rays, and of course, the actual crowns. He chose to ignore me.

The Subway Healings

▼

Replacing the toxic metals with benign materials required an additional three months time. Dr. Bellman followed the compatibility report, using only approved substances for my fillings, crowns, and adhesives for seating the crown. He sent me to an oral surgeon for the next procedures.

My root canal had to go. This decision went against Mom's dictum, and everything I had ever known about *keeping your teeth*, but I decided on the extraction based on Huggins's and other dentist's research, which showed that a root canal is a foreign body, sitting in the gum. A root canal, while having the appearance of a tooth, really for me was yet another unneeded assault on my immune system.

The tooth contained an old filling, and supported a crown with a high negative ammeter reading. The presence of this dead root made it a possible focus for anaerobic bacteria. Dr. Levin suggested I send the tooth to a lab involved in root canal research, at the University of Kentucky, and indeed it proved to be moderately toxic.

The successful surgery to remove the root canal tooth went well. In Huggins's text, I read about periodontal ligaments. These ligaments hold our teeth to the jaw, remain after most dental extractions, and can hold inflammatory lymphocytes. The periodontal ligament removal is a simple procedure designed to remove a source of assault on the immune system. I timed the extraction according to Dr. Bellman's ammeter readings, so it would simultaneously free me of the tooth with the root canal, its periodontal ligament and the crown with the high negative reading.

The suction noise intertwined with the squeaking sound coming from the root canal tooth as the oral surgeon eased it from the gum. Thanks to his local anesthetic, and a lovely assistant, I was comfortable. I slowly emerged from the building, my gum filled with local anesthesia. I was intent on getting home *before* the medication wore off.

It was not to be. I was about to be approached by four spirits, not all the same day, but yes, all for the same reason and therefore, interrelated.

The first spirit, who awaited me right after my surgery, was a raggedy, elderly woman, whose pasty face approached me as I inched toward the subway. Gray hair flying, she was erratically, and a bit loudly selling cards for the benefit of the Humane Society.

"Help a homeless cat, won't you?" she insisted.

Wordlessly, and without stopping, I handed her a dollar. She somehow blocked my path. "What's wrong?" she asked.

"Well," I retorted, without moving my jaw, which felt like it had grown to football proportions, "I'm recovering from a tooth extraction and if you'll excuse me, I'm going home before the pain gets extreme."

"So young to remove teeth…why?" she asked with assurance, as though she already knew.

"I have heavy metal toxicity; I got it from dental work," I replied through pursed lips.

"Dear, you need to listen to WBAI FM, that's 99.5. They discuss what can be done about that very subject."

"I'm a fellow listener!" I said, a bit incredulously, with wide-eyed attention.

"I recommend listening while drinking Mountain Valley mineral water in the green glass bottle. Confidentially, she whispered, you're going to bloom! Bloom, I tell you. Then, adopt a cat."

Only in New York, I thought, as I waved her goodbye at the subway entrance.

A few months later, I encountered the next *spirit* in the Eighth Avenue subway station, while on my way to the V.A. humor program. The E train crowd had thinned following morning rush hour. A black man wearing casual clothes and carrying a Bible, walked alongside me, stopping near the turnstile. "May I pray for you?" he asked kindly.

Now, when I think of prayer, I think of a serenely quiet, pleasant, activity. So, I smiled and said, "OK," stepping with my cane out of the path of the last commuters.

But when the *spirit* closed his eyes and opened his heart, his prayer was loud, as it fervently reverberated off the tunnel walls.

"Let my sister, Florence, be free of this illness," he boomed.

His Bible-holding hand wavered with the energy that surged through him, and coursed through my being, shaking me to the roots, flooding my heart with compassion.

I began to cry uncontrollably, so a woman stopped, and then a man, to ask anxiously whether I was all right. I looked around at the concerned faces of my fellow commuters, nodding yes, alternately laughing and crying. I had just experienced my first subway healing.

The prayers, first from the *Humane Society Spirit*, and then the African American preacher, so unexpected, so-out-of-church, were *touching* in a physical sense, like Healing Touch, that is, capable of moving energy through the power of love, in the form of goodwill.

The third spirit also came to me in a subway station, this time on the upper west side, after a chiropractic visit. I felt the usual good energy after my treatment; I was relaxed, energized, and calm. I stood with my cane, waiting for the next train, when a tall black man, shabbily dressed, and carrying a Bible, approached me. Why me? Was it the aluminum cane? It was as before, with a friendly stranger's desire to help. Did they attend the same church? Did they minister to all, or especially to people with canes on trains? These thoughts flew out of my mind as he began to pray. Looking up, I got a flash of his gums; he'd lost a few upper teeth.

"Jesus look down upon Sister Florence, and guide her toward healing. Protect and direct her life". Then the very tall man took both of my hands, putting *The Good Book* under his arm, and he shook my hands strongly, punctuating his prayer as the sweat poured from his face. Once again, tears flowed as if pulled from my throat, and with them, all my current frustration. My surprise sobs were muffled by the clatteringly approaching train, which I didn't notice. I felt my tears dissolve the pain of the all the falls I had taken, of all the confusion about the tests and therapies, and of mounting dental and chelation costs. The strange minister smiled, revealing lots of gaps, once occupied by front teeth. This time, a quietly curious crowd had gathered to be sure I was able to handle my second subway healing.

Prayer happens when the one prayed for is least aware. I suppose it also happens when a friend says, "Get home safely," or wishes you "Godspeed."

Six months passed. One windy day in autumn, I came out of my apartment with a cane. Wearing a backpack over my coat, under a bright blue sky, I was headed for the train station, and then to Pennsylvania, to visit my family. My heels and toes were my present focus as each slow step brought me the short block to the bus stop bench, where a tiny, brown-skinned woman sat, holding a shopping bag. She was elderly, with bright eyes that shone from under a knitted hat. I crept closer; each step measured and stabilized against the whipping wind by my new, precisely placed and faultless aluminum cane.

She watched me as I slowly sat on the bench. Then the little woman smiled excitedly, presenting me her gift, "I was praying…that you'd make it…to the bench." She was the fourth of the *spirits* who saw me through the year, 1998.

That year, I underwent three more chelation regimens. When I entered the office for the fourth one, something told me I wouldn't need it. I asked the technician to please phone the lab for my last metal reading.

"It's good," he said, smiling, as if describing a home run, one ear to the phone, "You're down to 1.6." At the start of this experiment, the mercury in the urine was too high to be measured, but then it dropped with each chelation. Escaping the now unnecessary chelation appointment, instead I celebrated by taking myself out for Indian food, and a movie, and felt very humored. After eight months, I was metal free, or so I assumed.

But I continued to be prone to spills. I gave up my daily T'ai chi practice, and my regular Yoga practice. My balance would no longer permit long lunges or backward movement, without a cane. Thanks to my lunch partner, that good old stand-by, WBAI, I learned Qi gong, when the radio station ran a daylong session with a Chinese master of that healing art.

He spoke of amazing recoveries he had seen in people who practiced the ancient exercise. In Essence Qi gong, I discovered the same benefits I had derived from T'ai chi, but without the tendency and risk of falling. The ancients devised a method of harmonizing energy by concentrating on the posture, and breath while repeating an exercise form.

I took the Qi gong session in the radio office, when it was located at Eighth Avenue and Thirty-Fifth streets, the nineteenth floor. I had a view of the tops of other skyscrapers out the window, as I waited in a line of fifty other listeners to register.

Taking my seat, I struck up a conversation with a man named Alex, who was a fellow listener, and Reiki master. Later, when we ate lunch, Alex would advise, "You're crossing your legs, and you know that short circuits chi." I uncrossed my legs, and then broke into a laugh as the master teacher, at the front of the room, as if on cue, crossed his.

The outdoor temperature was freezing, so I was rather uncomfortable, and off balance when we began. The Chinese master had a mission to teach all interested people about Qi gong, fueled by the success of his clients. A Chinese-American woman, who did the exercises, simultaneously translated his instructions. After an hour of practicing one of the exercise forms, I felt warmer and steadier. It was reassuring to me that the entire day's practice was done while safely standing, unlike the sweeping T'ai chi movements.

The three basic forms began with our energized hands facing the front of the body. The second form began with the hands facing the back of the body and the third addressed the sides of the body. We learned other forms, which released blocked chi from individual organs, beginning with the liver, and then the heart, the spleen, lungs, and finally, finishing with the kidneys.

I felt lighter by the end of the day when Genady met me. In rehashing the class with him, I decided that this twenty-minute workout would be a beneficial addition to my routine. Studying Qi gong gave me another unexpected benefit. I could clearly see the direct link that connected Chinese energy exercises, and Healing Touch therapy.

Speaking of exercise, and a feeling of well being, I had joined a weekly water aerobics program. In one hour's time, *Water aerobics* gave me energy, an aerobic workout, and the ability to do things I could not do on land, such as jogging in Speedo water shoes. Combined with a sauna, where perspiration released toxic wastes from the skin, I had flashes of being healthy.

There was humor in *Water aerobics*! I will never forget the sight of ten women plus Genady jogging in the pool to the pumping of the tune, *Where do I go?*, while they each held colorful Styrofoam noodles overhead. This exercise has a spark of childlike fun at its core. Other toys used to press against the water were barbells and webbed gloves.

1998

▼

At the start of 1998, I was practicing the following:
   Juicing with a vegetarian diet, including fish: three times each week.
   Qi gong: daily
   Nutritional supplements
   Tibetan herbs
   Meditation: sporadically
   Ayurvedic routines
   Panchakarma: every six months
   Water aerobics: once a week
   Humor
   IV chelation

Dream...
The Secret of Exhibit A
I'm in an apartment, expecting the police to visit; they search for clues to a crime. I'm worried. Detective Woody Allen enters, also worried, and I help him to calm down.
Daddy's old gray green navy trunk from the war is opened.
"Here is exhibit A," says the bespectacled detective, holding to the light an aged love letter, composed on fragile paper. "Oh, but the date is not significant," he adds, and I feel relieved. Then I see the trunk change into a shiny, electric blue suitcase.

Interpretation: the problem is transforming. Something good is happening. I have overcome the fear associated with this illness. The place in my heart, long forgotten, has been well remembered.

I was noticing speech improvements and less lethargy, but the balance prompted occasional falls. My energy wasn't much better, why was that? Perhaps most importantly, why did these comedians populate my dreams?

Dr. Levin has dropped a bomb on me. "You'll need more work to remove metal from the brain. The intravenous chelation doesn't cross the blood-brain barrier, so you'll need to do a challenge test with DMSA."

How stupid of me to celebrate so soon! Aren't the brain and the body connected? I guess only for humor therapy junkies. What is capable of crossing the blood-brain barrier is DMSA, (2,3 dimercaptosuccinic acid) a little white capsule, which I took late at night, six hours after my mineral supplements. This late night dose would prevent the metal chelator from pulling out important minerals. It also afforded me the benefit of chelation at home.

After six weeks of this routine, a challenge test was done: a large dose of DMSA chelate, followed by a six-hour collection of urine, to determine metal content. Hopefully it would hold successively fewer amounts of metal.

"Let us reclaim the body's terrain."

John Harris, WBAI producer of Urban Health Beat

About the same time that I began removing metals from my body, I started reacting to certain foods. The reaction usually took the form of abdominal pain, and diarrhea the following day. At Dr. Levin's urging, I tested for food allergies and learned that I had become allergic to about twenty foods. Among these were eggs, tomatoes, soy products, and wheat.

I went on a diet, devoid of the troublesome foods. A vegetarian for twenty-five years, I was able to stick to the regimen, although I found it nearly impossible to eat in a restaurant, and all processed food was out.

On advice from the Huggins Clinic, I chose to eat fish, which was ordered from my organic delivery service. They bought it from a place that raises fish in a healthy environment, uncontaminated by metals.

My diet also included daily grains, except for corn and wheat, lots of green and yellow vegetables, and occasional fruit. I increased my intake of good fats such as flax, and olive oil, to help protect nerve tissue, to add fuel, and to avoid having my stored fat burned as calories. From my experience with Ayurveda, I included sea salt with the trace minerals left intact, and spices, such as turmeric to support my immune system.

But after two years, I was beginning to tire of the restricted diet, which kept me at a scant one hundred five pounds. The word diet begins with die. Not that I died, but my higher carbohydrate diet of the past, died. Though my body was indeed reedy, there was something tree-like about my spirit. I mused, as to whether it was a result of T'ai chi's exercise, *holding the tree*.

I read an article on the Natural Allergy Elimination Treatment, in the spring issue of *New Age* magazine. The treatment uses muscle testing, and a sort of marriage between massage, and acupuncture. Muscle testing involves holding the offending allergen, as the practitioner attempts to move one of the patient's arms. If there is solid resistance, it indicates no allergy. If the arm is weak enough to fall, this is an indication of allergy. NAET reeducates the brain about allergens so that it doesn't automatically identify the good nutrients in food, as offenders to be reacted against.

"Holy Tofu!" I exclaimed, as I read the article, "My digestion could be normal again!"

NAET works in part, by changing what the body views as an allergen. Instead of targeting, say, a tomato, NAET prohibits the brain from having an allergic reaction to the Vitamin C in tomatoes, and in other foods. I would locate an NAET practitioner.

I pushed through yet another huge glass door on Forty-Second and Madison Avenue, thanks to a doorman who should get an award for hospitality. He could have been a lineman, but instead, he intercepts elevators for me, and smiles.

The mahogany desk of Dr. Jean Miller's seventeenth floor office was completely clear, except for her phone, pad, and pen. She admitted that how NAET works is still partly a mystery.

"Theories. Just theories," she said softly, as she placed a vial of the first allergen, egg, in my hand. I lay on a treatment table, and she used the opposite arm for the muscle test; surely, I was allergic to eggs. Then she cleared the energy centers, by moving her hands in front of my body for a half-minute, like Healing Touch technique. Face down on the treatment table, I received a spinal massage on the muscles of my back, using a set of Bongers; oversized, spongy drumsticks much like the type used to play the xylophone. I finally turned face up, as acupuncture needles were inserted at points such as the web of the hand, the elbow, the area below the knee, and the top of the foot. The acupuncture needles are so fine that there is no pain involved: in fact the procedure was pleasant! For the treatment to process, I was told to relax for twenty minutes. This was a deliciously restful time, in that dimly lit, quiet space, with Jean's soft music, and the needles helping to move the chi.

"Remember now, don't eat eggs for twenty-four hours," she said in parting, "and then, try an omelet."

My eyes shot open. What? After years of an egg less diet, I whipped up an omelet, mostly to see what my body would have to say about it. I excitedly sautéed onion, tossing in fresh basil, and parsley at the end for a filling. Rice would accompany the main course.

When my body responded with *bon-appetite*, I scheduled my visits to Jean Miller every week, after the V.A. humor group. They were the most pleasant doctor visits I ever had, not only because they followed good humor, and were in a pleasant office, but also because, one-by-one, all the allergens were eliminated, from eggs to soy, and from mushrooms to metals.

According to Dr. Miller, I had become allergic to many metals, and during the twenty-four hour processing period after the NAET metal clearing, I was instructed to wear gloves, so that I wouldn't touch metal. In addition, NAET allowed me to up my intake of Vitamin C. With more of the antioxidant in my diet, my immune system would be stronger. About this time, I eliminated all sugar except for the occasional fruit treat.

Jean Miller intended to improve my balance, and spoke positively about it each week, as she did the spinal massage phase of my treatment.

While my balance was unaffected by NAET, I decided to give myself more insurance against falls, and bought a walker with large wheels, and bicycle-like hand brakes. I could move safely, go faster, and carry heavy items in its basket, which freed me to shop, without having to drop. This red, wheeled machine, I named, *The Device.*

Nine months after I began NAET, my allergy symptoms had cleared up. Eggplant, and certain types of pepper could bring on symptoms, but I could eat almost anything I really wanted. I could even dine in a restaurant! I had come to trust a few places that served healthy fare, but now, with my stronger digestive ability, I could venture into unknown establishments on a vacation. My frame slowly filled out as proof of better absorption of nutrients. We celebrated at Angelica's Kitchen, a vegan restaurant, in the East Village. Angelica, I learned, was an herb, related to the carrot family, which in the Middle Ages, was credited with neutralizing diseases such as the plague. Because my husband was on a low-cholesterol diet, he liked the spot on Twelfth Street, and there were no dairy foods in the recipes. I enjoyed the way they took vegetables, and turned them safely into gourmet feasts. The entrance of Angelica's has a blackboard on which a quote of the day was written:

> The snow goose
> need not bathe
> to make itself white.
> Neither need you
> do anything
> but be yourself
> Lao-tse

On the restaurant walls were painted Geordian knots, lighted by sconce-held candles. We waited in a short line to be seated, by a local student from NYU. She recommended the special on today's menu: Bravetart, a baked concoction of sweet potatoes, and other root veggies. Whoever was in charge of naming these dishes certainly had a sense of humor, naming them after movies and sports heroes. We started with their famed *pate*, which did look and taste like foie de gras, but was made of lentils. We enjoyed our entrees in the lively company of other vegetarians, and finished our meal over grain coffee, plus a small slice of chocolate torte, a decadently dense cake made with soy. Although it was not a small dinner, we noticed that our stomachs felt very light.

Bodywork and Supportive Therapies

▼

Panchakarma, with its attendant bodywork, taught me to pay more attention to my body. I began to get more therapeutic massage, in an effort to wring out the offending metals. I learned that massage goes way beneath the muscle. *Hands-on* therapies go all the way to the bones. Over the years, many therapists had helped with this restorative activity, but the one who affected me long after the one-hour session, was Anthony Brancale.

He was a graduate of the Edgar Cayce School, and later learned to drain lymphatic fluid. Lots of waste products leave the tissues via lymph channels, which having no pump, depend upon exercise, deep breaths, and yes, laughter, to drain these impurities.

The average person has about twelve quarts of lymph, a sort of irrigation system, going at all times. Composed of water and used nutrients, its stagnation can lead to pain and low energy, not to mention blocked lymph nodes. The branches of the lymph system parallel the circulatory system, with its tree-like roots below the neck, the trunk at the base of the neck with the thoracic duct, which is where lymphatic fluid empties into the venous circulation. Lymph channels from the entire body drain into the thoracic duct.

Massage is an excellent adjunct to the body's usual avenues of lymph drainage, releasing energy blockages. With his clairvoyant abilities, Cayce was known for a multitude of healing successes. For example, the abdominal heat pack recommended by Scott Gerson, was identical to the one in the Cayce readings.

Anthony's technique of lymphatic drainage opened the trunk portion of the lymph tree, moving lymph fluid by massage throughout the body, carrying toxins to the veins in the elimination process. Lymphatic drainage was also addressed in Janet Mentgen's Healing Touch course I had taken. I also practice her drainage technique, which I found stimulating to skin and nerves.

Anthony wisely taught me how to clean lymph from the throat, which helped me to swallow, and to speak clearly. Massaging the throat with both hands, I could open the lymph trunk. Then with my thumb, I rubbed the soft palate, which produced a fair amount of clear fluid, indistinguishable from saliva. While doing this routine one morning, I wondered whether my overabundant saliva might partially be lymphatic fluid just trying to clear? I found immediate benefits for speech, swallowing and energy when I did this practice. It was another reminder to me of the body's quietly expedient powers.

Since exercise moves lymph, I incorporated the *bouncing ball* that I used in physical therapy. I would ride this in winter, when I would rather not go outside, yet needed the exercise. Sitting on my large, blue exercise ball gave me the benefits of a trampoline, without injury. Since I had heard on WBAI radio, that marches are good for nerve integration, I played Sousa or the "1812 Overture," used for the series, *The Lone Ranger* (rides again).

At first my feet slid out from my sitting position on the air-filled bouncing ball, but the problem was solved when I pulled on my rubber pool shoes for traction. Look Ma, no hands! Hi-ho Silver, away!

The brain and the ear are connected. Music therapy for me has meant medieval chants on Sunday morning, Indian ragas for giving or receiving massage, Tibetan wind instrumentation for soaking in the tub, early Elvis when doing laundry, and man, does Beatle music cook! Bob Marly's full-of-life-rhythm is wedded to poetry. I get dressed, often listening to Bob sing, "Every little thing gonna be all right." Another auditory tonic to me is the voice of sweet baby James Taylor. I have thought maybe it's the words, maybe the soothing tone, but in the end it just is the right frequency for my ear.

The comedy team performing *Monty Python's* music is the funniest, and is ideal for drive time. Replaying it hundreds of times has not diminished the frequency or amplitude of our resulting belly laughs. One of their best tunes is *I'm so worried, worried, worried.*

The musical geniuses, Marly, and the Pythons in particular, have endeared themselves to me because they stare down every monster, from travel anxiety to death, obliterating all with the power of laughter, and the wisdom of humor.

I could not leave the ear as an avenue of healing, without mentioning a therapy called Bioacoustics; the study of the frequencies produced by all living systems. One day, my friend Trudy called to say she had heard of a sound therapy that was a cross between music therapy, and biofeedback.

This discussion led me to have my voice analyzed, because by *printing* the voice, Bioacoustics is able to detect health issues, and then treat them using sound. I had to take another journey in order to create my voice prescription, a two-hour ride on a NJ Transit train, to The Davis Center, in Budd Lake, New Jersey. There I was greeted by a trio of autistic children, who were there for another type of sound therapy. The Bioacoustitian, Glenora Broadwell, was an L.P.N., who quickly demonstrated her knowledge of sounds as they relate to health.

Handing me a microphone, she coached, "Speak normally into this and I'll tell you when to stop." Soon after I spoke, I saw my voice mapped on the screen of her laptop computer.

"The lines remind me of an EKG," I observed.

"Now, you take a seat outside," said Glenora, "while I feed the voice print into the computer. I'll take from the print very low, and very high tones. These will reflect certain deficiencies in your body. Then we make a tape for you to listen to every day. The object of this is to normalize brain waves, to help the body eliminate toxins, better utilize nutrients, and strengthen your muscles."

I thought this deserved a try because it was noninvasive, had helped others with neurological symptoms, and it cost me less than some doctor visits. The first three months of listening to the therapeutic tones, I had no falls! None. This was reason to continue. The second session of printing revealed to Glenora that positive changes had occurred in my brain. She took the previous sound formula, refining it for more balance. I would continue going for Bioacoustic voice printing and sound prescriptions three times each year. The sounds were soothing low tones that became part of my meditation routine. The prints revealed successively fewer toxins, normalizing as years went by.

One day while I practiced Qi gong in the empty office waiting room of Dr. Levin, I struck up a conversation with Michael, a medical technician, who had gone to acupuncture school.

"You know, if you're trying to dislodge a boulder, it takes patience, and tools just to get it to roll. Think of yourself as building chi against this object. The hard part is in the dislodging. Acupuncture, done by one with experience, can benefit chronic illness," he declared.

He gave me the number of a Chinese doctor in Queens, and I resumed acupuncture after a two-year hiatus. Dr. Ping Fu, a young woman with long black hair, which she said was long and black, thanks to eating black sesame seed, had twenty years of experience practicing her craft in New York, California, and China. Her father had been a renowned acupuncturist in China.

Her chi was boundless. Determined, without being overbearing, she was a one-woman band who answered the door, inserted the needles, dispensed herbs, and did the billing. A far cry from the usual doctor's office, I thought, while I sipped her *Dragonwell* green tea.

Dr. Fu checked my pulse before and during the treatment. She peered into my mouth, to see my tongue. My tongue told her that the chi needed support, as many treatments as possible. That meant once weekly. Daily

Qi gong would suffice on the other six days. When I inquired about the pulse diagnosis, I wasn't surprised when she referred to the problem as a *wind imbalance*. Dr. Dhonden's herbs had treated the wind component. Ayurvedic pulse diagnosis referred to it as an over abundant vata (air) element, and deficient pitta (fire) element.

Dr. Fu proceeded to place almost every one of her forty plus needles in the back of my body. She felt that the spine and brain would determine the ability of the body to recover. My previous encounter with the ancient treatment had all been anterior, and had involved about a dozen of the needles. She also attached a nerve stimulator to spinal points.

Although she told me that it would be a slow process, the effect of acupuncture on my energy was evident after the first month's treatment. I accomplished my activities more quickly and easily. I seemed to have halted the worsening of my neurological symptoms. Yes, there were occasional falls, and walking remained difficult, but my voice was close to normal within a year. Sporadic aches and pains sustained from minor injuries, usually disappeared after a few treatments.

After dedicating myself to receiving acupuncture for several months, I was convinced of its positive effects on my body and mind. More than that, I began to feel energy differently in people, food, inanimate objects, and in the way I viewed the world.

1999

1999 routines included:
- Qi gong: daily
- Energy work
- Water aerobics and sauna: three days per week
- Tibetan herbs, Chinese herbs
- Nutritional supplements
- Oral chelation
- Bodywork: about monthly
- NAET: weekly
- Acupuncture: weekly
- Panchakarma: every six months
- Chiropractic: every other month
- Self applied lymphatic drainage: at least 4 days per week
- Bioacoustics
- Humor

Dream…

Lifelike, was that dreaming? I ride in the back of a van with Christina Gerson. We're wearing these elegant, warm, winter hats, as we depart from a Panchakarma retreat. There are other participants in the vehicle, but the only recognizable face is Chris Farley, comedian of *Saturday Night Live*. As I write this, I recall that his *motivational speaker* character lived in a van. Maybe the van belonged to him, but on with the dream.

I jumped out of the van at a station of some kind. I walk with perfect balance and coordination, so natural that I don't even notice, and then I suddenly recall the cane and the walker device. But I don't need them as I walk with a new sureness to the basement elevator and go UP.

I find Honey in a sort of airport lounge. He comes out and my ecstatic story spills out. He smiles, saying, "Yes."

Interpretation: a view of the future.

I began 1999 with my Ayurvedic routine of deep winter: increased rest. Basically, I adhered to the same regimen as in 1998. I continued Qi gong practice, which calmed me, and although my symptoms remained consistent, I also took the metal chelating agent. I was able to walk for miles with the device or walker, provided I didn't do it too often.

Dr. Fu prescribed many herbs to strengthen the yang. Yang is the Chinese term for active, advancing energy. Yang is the opposite of yin or receding energy. The herbal formula did not seem to have an obvious effect until she added Korean Ginseng to the herbal compound, in the summer of 1999. When the supplier ran out of the formula, my chi dropped significantly. I tried to find it in the health food store, but had no luck.

I reminded Dr. Fu about this several times. One day she offered me a high-grade of powdered Korean Ginseng. It was more than a tonic. Overnight I began to want to do more energy intensive activities, like workout in the pool. I took it first thing in the morning to rev me up for the day's activities, and then again at dinner, to support cellular repair at night. Why such a dramatic effect from Ginseng? I did some research and found that there could be a combination of reasons. It enhances immunity, and supports the adrenal glands, which relates to our ability to handle stress. It also contains vitamins A, B1, B12, and E.

The year 1999, proved to be my most difficult, for I would need increased energy on the emotional as well as the physical level. My mother had reached the age of eighty-three, and was no longer able to care for herself. She had a form of geriatric diabetes, and my sister, Cindy was interested in keeping close tabs on her blood sugar. The house in which we spent our childhood was too much work for an elderly woman, and plans were made to move her to the home of my sister, and brother-in-law. Mom's memory was growing dimmer, which made it especially important that medicine and meals were not forgotten. Due to this memory deficit, she communicated with us, but remembered very little of what was said. Our life-long habit of chats, seasoned with humor, had become a thing of the past. Mom, my humor model, had embodied Norman Cousins' definition of humor, with love, faith, festivity, and determination as well as laughter.

At the same time, in addition to his computer-oriented work, Genady was being given a job opportunity to do the work of a lifetime. He had earned his scuba diving instructor status, and was offered jobs in Florida, and Pennsylvania, which would mean regular weekend, or longer, trips away from home. I felt in my own heart the importance attached to his job opportunity, yet pulled by Mom, and distanced from Genady, I felt trapped in an emotional tug-of-war.

Genady stood with me in front of the turquoise ocean in Mexico. He was there to work, while I was on vacation. It all hit me one morning before he left on the dive boat, to guide his scuba group. I held the walker handles steadily, but my voice wavered.

"I feel such incredible sadness," I said to Genady. "First Mom's troubles…that I felt were straining enough. Now I'll be seeing you less than I do now…it's separation anxiety."

"I'm not leaving *you*," he said with feeling, "I'm following my heart's desire…it's kind of like giving birth…"

I answered, "I know it's a big achievement, to do what feeds your soul."

In reality, I knew he wanted to do scuba training as a full-time job, so I supported his dream, as he had been so supportive of mine. The adjustment to his work schedule was difficult, but I managed to adapt by searching for the humor in my situation, and by using the quantity of free time available to me for the completion of this book.

Humor will always surface. I knew that when you most need it, it's most elusive, so I turned to my spiritual leader, Swami Beyondananda.

The wise one started by admonishing me, in a pseudo Indian accent, for not getting rid of that toxic car.

"But Swami, I never owned a Mercury," I reminded him.

He seemed surprised. "Stand on your head. It keeps unwanted thoughts from trickling down into the body. Sounds as though you could use a mental flossing. Let painful thoughts go in one ear, with the floss, and out the other! Enlighten up while you're at it."

His advice was perfect, for laughs. I never could stand on my head, let alone today. I actually reverted to his *Tantrum Yoga*. I did it on my way to exercise. I stomped my foot as though I were as large as King Kong, toppling buildings in my wake. The buildings were my problems.

This emotional trial induced me to do something I had longed to do for years. I signed up for a weekend course in the use of Bach Flower Essences. It has since proved to be an indispensable component to my healing.

The British Dr. Edward Bach, originated this method in the thirties. He prepared flowers in a manner similar to homeopathy. "Human emotional states could be treated by using specific flowers," he had said, "to gain a peaceful equilibrium." Actually, flower remedies work on the emotional layer of the human aura, which in a stagnant state, can aggravate physical ailments. I related to Dr. Bach's philosophy of treating the patient, not the disease, and began using a variety of flowers, to treat my emotional tug-of-war. A month later I felt as though a weight the size of an anvil had dropped off my body.

I knew the most renowned of the essences, Rescue Remedy, but knew little about the other thirty-eight. I began to rely on Rescue Remedy for the previously described dental visits. It is intended to treat any degree of emotional stress, so I began keeping it in my purse, in case of emergency.

Six months after I started making flower formulas for myself, I felt more like the old Florence, even laughing more. According to my instructor, Elizabeth Wylie, happiness is a possible side effect of Bach treatments, but peace was what Dr. Bach intended.

Long distance transmissions

▼

One spring day, Genady's aunt, who lived in Israel, phoned to recommend a *Naturopathic* practitioner named Valentina, who spoke only in Russian. She urged taking a chance on a different form of energy.

"She has the ability to work long distance," Genady's Aunt Netta said, "She can transmit energy for healing from her home to yours, thousands of miles away." Genady agreed to phone and translate my situation to Valentina.

Valentina asked to speak to me so she could hear my voice; the quality of it. Through Aunt Netta, I understood that she wanted me to mail her a photo, and to try the method for one week before deciding whether or not I wanted to work with her. After all, she admitted, some people don't relate to long distance healing. Although I had never had an *official* healing session, from a practitioner in a remote location, I remembered that Manny Cline had sent me a form of this energy work from his office to my home. I decided to try long-distance healing.

Valentina prescribed herbal teas, to clear toxins, and metals. I located a local naturopath, and herbalist, at Angelica's Herbs, on Ninth and First Avenue, whose shop was a cornucopia of leaves, powders, and blossoms. A sign on the wall cautioned: NO TAPING OR PHOTOGRAPHS PLEASE.

To my surprise, Chantal, the owner, had also experienced heavy metal toxicity, recovering through the use of herbs and juicing. Her clientele, I discovered, was a patiently loyal group, often waiting in line a good half-hour for a particular cream, tea, or incense.

While serving me one day, she threw a few grains of bee pollen in her mouth, and said with a French accent, "I'm on my feet all day, I need an energy boost." Then filling a small brown paper bag with my bee pollen, she told me, "This'll keep safely in the fridge for six months, inside a plastic bag."

She tended to agree with Valentina's prescription, often suggesting additional cleansing products.

"Good that you're taking Laminaria. You can add a spoon of it to bath water, and then add this clay," she pointed to a jar of gray clay for facials, "to soak out impurities."

As had become my custom, an honest trial would be done: that being the only means of knowing, in my case, whether the herbs had restorative qualities.

The herbs were intriguing to read about, and to use. Calm seemed to exude from the leaves and flowers in a refreshing way. To mention a few of these herbs: Sage, as a nerve tonic, Nettle, as a cleansing agent, Yarrow, as an appetite stimulant, and anti-inflammatory agent, and Red Clover to support immunity. The Laminaria would assist in the elimination of metal, and the energy boosting bee pollen would be most welcome.

Valentina planned her energy transmissions for late evening, and gave me the following instructions. Four days each week, at the appointed time of three P.M., my time, I would say a prayer, light a candle, and take a glass of water to the bedroom, where I was to lie still for an hour. I began to feel a sensation, a vibration, about five minutes later. Then I always fell asleep! Was I so exhausted? I wondered. I usually did not feel tired. Stranger still, I would awaken as the hour ended, rarely continuing to sleep.

The water, present during the energy transmission, was now also *charged* with energy, and I was instructed to drink it, following the session. I agreed to do this routine for a month at a time, as the per-session cost of ten dollars, was reasonable. I had an almost immediate abatement of the few nagging food allergy symptoms, which remained after NAET.

After three months of long distance healing, and Chantal's herbs, in the autumn of 1999, I discontinued the process. Evidence in the form of mercury testing reflected the value of the long-distance energy work: my level of mercury had dropped to *trace levels*. This indicates that there is some of the metal, but not enough to measure. My walking remained uncoordinated, although I was enjoying walks of up to three miles. My balance, a continual tightrope act, responded to my health practices. The ginseng prescribed by Dr. Fu, fueled my activities. The sweat poured from me, after only ten minutes in the pool sauna. Pulse diagnoses of Dr. Gerson, and Dr. Fu, proved I had a much different body than the body I had taken to the neurologist!

2000

▼

As one Millennium ended, and a new one began, my health routine had expanded to include:
Acupuncture: weekly
Qi gong: daily energy exercise
Water aerobics and sauna: three times per week
Organic diet, supplemented by vitamins, minerals and juiced vegetables
Bodywork: about every month
Panchakarma: every six months
Bach Flower remedies
Homeopathic remedies
Daily meditation
Bioacoustics
Humor

A lucid dream…
An imposing and menacing woman with blonde, rope-like braids, comes at me head on. She's in a Nordic operatic costume, minus the typical horned helmet.
From within the clouds of my sleep, I knew it to be a dream. "She represents the disease," I thought as I halted my escape and chose to take complete control. I started to close in on the threatening operatic monster, saying, "GET OUT." I took hold of it. It felt hot, melting for a second before it transformed. I was overjoyed to see that it became my plush

blond dog, Puppy. Puppy was a sweet and friendly dog of mine from years ago, a dog that had made it his work to protect me.

Heavy metal disease has assaulted my nerves, my muscles, interrupted my digestion, and wreaked havoc on my ability to sleep, but it won't kill me, not as long as I keep my health as the highest priority.

Belief in this body, has served to pull me through many dark hours. Help had come from practitioners who knew the importance of surrounding their patients with positive energy, and convincing them to keep trying. It has been said that when anyone experiences healing, it leads to the healing of others. My restored energy makes it possible for me to adhere to the routines I have listed by the year. My humor therapy group work has expanded. Through the Healing Works Foundation, in New York, I've been privileged to laugh with groups who work to care for people with HIV, abused children, and the elderly.

I continue to walk with *The Device,* or a cane. My voice shows continual improvement along with my energy. From the nightmarish start of this adventure, my body responded to almost any prudent attempt to nurture it, provided I didn't expect overnight results.

What is the value of this journey? I recently answered this question for a friend, joking that the only redeeming value is in the free bus rides provided by a certain bus driver. I have become a humble student of the world, the Earth, and its inhabitants. The continual opportunities to learn from this body are invaluable, as it teaches me that it is all I really have, and so must be given priority. I have learned to love the uncertainty, while refusing to fit into the picture that is offered by closed minded practitioners. While I have a flexible time schedule compared to the days of working in the hospital, most of my time is devoted to healing practices.

Perhaps it is all about relaxation. I knew that humor and laughter brought about *release and relaxation,* but so do most of the practices listed as my self-created prescriptions!

2002

▼

My healthcare prescription includes:
- Bikram Yoga
- Panchakarma: every six months
- Organic diet with supplements
- Qi gong: twice weekly
- Daily meditation
- Bioacoustics daily
- Bodywork: monthly
- Homeopathic remedies
- Bach Flower remedies
- Tricycle riding: two or three times weekly in good weather
- Humor

Homeopathic remedies help eliminate toxins, and add energy. Metals were in the air from the fumes of the World Trade Center disaster, affecting many New Yorkers. I was no exception, and I dealt with it through the above regime, to which I added Laminaria, a sea vegetable, and pulverized Chlorella, a metal eliminating form of algae, which is chlorophyll. I was overdue for a holiday from my many supplements. Stopping them about every six weeks to take a week off did not appear to adversely affect my condition. As the year ends, I have eliminated all but basic dietary supplements. My nutritional education continues. Energy is improving also because I am more conscious about the energy that my food provides. Fresh fruits and vegetables always give me the best energy boost. I have also come to realize my own body needs more protein than I received when I was younger and in better health.

My vision of riding a bicycle has become reality. When Genady and I moved to New Jersey, I decided not to wait for my balance to improve before I rode that bike in the real live, out-of-doors. Therefore, the bike became trike! Within the excitement of fast locomotion, a tricycle eliminates my problem of balancing on wheels, strengthens muscles, and provides physical humor therapy! I actually belly laugh while triking! So do the people who pass me for the first time.

Exercising the legs, and perspiring, is beneficial to the cardiovascular system. I know my brain likes doing these movements so fluidly. Sunshine clears cobwebs from my head, and nature gives me perspective. Lymph channels clear with exercise, so I accomplish a lot of good for a little effort on the trike; the same benefits I previously sought with such diligence.

This playful device is an ageless symbol of freedom. People have been staring at me ever since I began using a cane. "They're just curious," my nephew, Matt, told me. When I ride the trike, I'm liberated from being a curiosity. Now I'm playing, just finding the fun.

Humoring the Patient When the Patient is Me

▼

"If you saw your problems on a stage in a play by Neil Simon, you would laugh yourself right out of your chair."

Louise Hay

Humor is my strength. A great body of research supports the value of humor as a vehicle for relaxation, and for the release of anxiety. When I faced the neuromuscular disease crisis, I really embarked on a mission that offered little assurance, and no guarantees. I was to learn that more regular doses of humor helped me to cope with it, and strengthened my general mental health. I recalled patients who had triumphed over serious illnesses, and resolved to learn how I could, too.

I treated myself to funny books, *feel good* movies, and I involved myself with laugh groups dedicated to humor. My schedule became less exacting, and I noticed even more humor in my surroundings when I stopped to smell the roses. The strength came to try new approaches to health, facing down any fear. It was as though risking the personal and public use of humor, made all risks less risky. I treated intense frustrations by sitting still, and then laughing (usually at a videotape) as soon as possible. I saw new delights in old videos. Steve Martin, as *The Jerk*, saved my sanity many a dark, winter night.

I became more loving toward myself, and, in turn, toward everyone around me. The thought occurred to me that in using and experiencing humor, I was also tapping into a love connection. *Applying* humor opens the heart. When one is dedicated enough to *self-apply* humor consistently, it is possible to love yourself, and others more deeply.

What an awareness of humor creates is a way for us to enjoy ourselves in the moment. We are better able to laugh at ourselves. When we attempt to invite humor, most of the time, life just seems to love us more. We find more enjoyment in our seeking it, and then we attract like-minded souls to this peaceful place.

My education in humor therapy began with a personal need for positive emotion. I read about the effects of laughter on the cardiovascular and respiratory systems. Then I contemplated how the surgical nurse must encourage post-operative patients to do deep breathing exercises, and saw a correlation for humor in the hospital. Further study of the positive effect of humor on the immune system, and for enhanced communication in therapy, convinced me to try to employ it at the bedside of the hospitalized patient.

Although I am not a comedian, I joked successfully with select patients, and also made a hit by using funny toys like Groucho Marx glasses. I found that patients relaxed and communicated more openly, and that they humored me in return. I saw that my own work stress seemed to be less when I consciously used humor, perhaps because I ceased to be victimized by the demands of the management or the patients.

Perhaps the most important thing I learned while using humor at the bedside of hospitalized patients was that my own genuine sense of humor, in becoming more visible, helped the patient.

I took uplifting humor into a darker place: the treatment center for veterans of the armed services, who had become homeless drug and alcohol addicts. This time I did it as a volunteer. In the beginning, I wanted to find out whether people who were in the throes of the biggest life-change, that of recovery from negatively addicting substances, could benefit by a positive addiction to humor. The answer was a resounding YES! I witnessed the change after only fifteen minutes of group laughter. Even seriously depressed men on the outside of our meeting room, were smiling. I encouraged the learning of jokes, prop play with funny glasses, and other clown disguises. This set the stage for the sharing of personal humorous encounters the men had while living in the streets.

A great gift of joy surfaced in the homeless humor sessions. I went there many times with little energy of my own. I would convince myself to act well enough to persuade just one person to laugh with me, and most of the time, the spirit within the group pulled us all above our problems. We acted as though we were well.

The men forgot their pain within their willingness to play.

The professional nurse groups who called me to do presentations, as well as the homeless veterans, enjoyed playing comedian by practicing improvisational humor. Improv is a great exercise in building group cohesion while empowering the individual. I emphasized combining emotion, any emotion, with humor. The groups often experienced a deep sense of release. Concurrently, they appeared so funny that I had to remark that the only difference between their performance and that of real actors was that the actors received a paycheck.

The most important thing I learned by doing improvisation was that group involvement is where the magic happens. Anyone, even the shyest person, can become a comedian! We accomplish this with the support of the group.

I have elaborated on the beauty of laughter clubs. The most important thing I learned in the laughing club sessions is that it required even less work on my part. The group spirit did the work. Laughing became easier, not only in the session, but at any other humorous time. More than that, I had the grateful feeling that finally someone, Dr. Kataria, had found a way to motivate the Earth's inhabitants to seek out humor therapy.

Iren Bischofberger, a nurse and specialist in humor therapy, enlightened me on the feeling state associated with humor. We led a group of

Swiss nurses in a study of humor therapy and laughter. Someone began a debate on the difference between humor and joy. After a long, funny discussion, we decided that joy is a kind of supercharged form of peace. Humor is the raw material of joy.

Perhaps because I'm better grounded due to an intense focus on my body, I find more of this joy infusing me. My perspective is clearer, which makes problems more easily solved.

Illness has been a strict taskmaster; necessitating new diets, sleep schedules, and exercises. But it breeds a form of creative thinking that evolved by the intention to improve my health. Using humor in my outlook, and observation of everyday life has created a stronger resolve, and reassurance about the future.

Now, with compromised health, I need humor more than any other medicine. Laughs are feeding my soul while lifting me over obstacles. The steadfast belief that humor is a necessity has prompted me to continue sharing laughter with others. Regardless of how often I laugh in group settings, I discover new pleasure, new wisdom, and new levels of release. Humor is energy!

I will never forget October 31, 1999, the day I learned I was free of metals. I had gone to Dr. Levin's office. While the lab technician took a blood specimen from my arm, I casually glanced at the sheet of lab results on my chart. Written there were the words: MERCURY TRACE.

With bated breath I asked, "Are you sure it's my chart?"

"It's yours," said the robot-like technician, monotonously. She did not have any idea that for five years of my life I had sweat, slept, and dieted, intent upon detoxification. I had relentlessly followed a tortuous, mercurial path, which had taken me through many heavy metal doors, and into the presence of gifted healers. A new path, freer of metals, opened for me on that day. I felt she was talking about my life: "It's yours."

References

Ayurveda:
Gerson, Scott. *Ayurveda: The Ancient Indian Healing Art.* Brewster, New York: National Institute for Ayurvedic Medicine, 1993.
Tiwari, Maya. *A Life of Balance.* Rochester, Vermont: Healing Arts Press, 1995.

Cookbooks:
Gates, Donna, and Linda Schatz. *The Body Ecology Diet.* Atlanta, Georgia: B.E.D. Publications, 1996.
Morningstar, Amadea, and Urmila Desai. *Ayurvedic Cookbook.* Wilmot, Wisconsin: Lotus Press, 1990.
Rigg, Jaque C. *Curing the Incurable.* Seattle, Washington: Hara Publishing, 1999.

Holistic Dentistry:
Briener, Mark A. *Whole Body Dentistry.* Fairfield, Connecticut: Quantum Health Press, 1999.
Huggins, Hal A. 1993. *It's All in Your Head.* Garden City Park, New York: Avery.
Kennedy, David C. *How to Save your Teeth.* Health Action Press, 1993.
Levy, Thomas E. *Detoxification After Dental Revision.* Videotape. Colorado Springs, Colorado: Peak Energy Performance, Inc. 4/ 19/1997.

Humor Therapy:
Bhaerman, Steve. *Driving Your own Karma*. Rochester, Vermont: Destiny Books, 1989.
Bhaerman, Steve. *When You See a Sacred Cow, Milk It For All It's Worth*. Lower Lake, California: Aslan Publishing, 1993.
Buxman, Karyn. *Nursing Perspectives on Humor*. Staten Island, New York: Power Publications, 1995.
Cousins, Norman. *Head First-The Biology of Hope*. New York, New York: Dutton, 1989.
Gesell, Izzy. *Playing Along: 37 Activities Borrowed from Improvisational Theater*. Duluth, Minnesota: Whole Person Associates, 1997.
Metcalf, C.W., and Roma Flelible. *Lighten Up*. Reading, Massachusetts: Addison-Wesley, 1992.
Wooten, Patty. *Compassionate Laughter*. Salt Lake City, Utah: Commune-A-Key Publishing, 1996.

Energy Studies:
Bruyere, Rosalyn L. *Wheels of Light*. New York: Simon and Schuster, 1989.
Choudry, Bikram. *Bikram Yoga*. New York, New York: Tarcher/Putnam Publishers, 2000.
Rhee, Jhoon. *Shim Shin Key*. Alexandria, VA: Time-Life Video, 1995. Videotape.

Nutrition:
Balch, James F. M.D. and Balch, Phyllis C.N.C. *Prescription for Nujtritional Healing*. Garden City Park, New York: Avery, 1997.

Spiritual Enhancement:
Marciniak, Barbara. *Earth*. Santa Fe, New Mexico: Bear & Co., 1995.

Video Humor Selections:

Aykroyd, Dan. *Doctor Detroit.* Universal City, California: MCA Home Video, 1983.

Breckman, Andy. *Rat Race.* Hollywood, California: Paramount Pictures, 2002.

Cleese, John. *A Fish Called Wanda.* New York, New York: CBS/FOX Video, 1989.

Dangerfield, Rodney. *It's not Easy Bein' Me.* New York, New York: Orion Home Video, 1987.

Martin, Steve. L.A. Story. Van Nuys, California: LIVE Home Video, 1991.

Martin, Steve. Mixed Nuts. Culver City, California: Columbia Tristar Home Video, 1995.

Martin, Steve. The Jerk. Universal City, California: MCA Home Video, 1991.

Monty Python's. And Now For Something Completely Different. Burbank, California: RCA/Columbia Pictures Home Video, 1991.

Monty Python's. *The Meaning of Life.* Universal City, California: MCA Home Video, 1996.

Python Pictures. Monty Python and the Holy Grail. Burbank, California: RCA/Columbia Pictures Home Video, 1991.

Ramis, Howard. Groundhog Day. Burbank, California: RCA/Columbia Pictures Home Video, 1993.

Reiner, Carl: Oh, God! Burbank, California: Warner Home Video, 1983.

Shapiro, Ken. *The Groove Tube.* Los Angeles, California: Media Home Entertainment, 1981.

Winters, Jonathan. Gone Fish'n. Nashville, Tennessee: Good Time Fish'n Video Company, 1993.

Word Index

Acupuncture, 4, 9-10, 85-86, 115-116, 122-124, 131
Adams, Patch, 30
Adler, Joseph, 36-37
Allergies, 114
American Association for Applied and Therapeutic Humor, 20, 29-30, 32
American Holistic Nurses Association, 58, 86-87
Amyotropic Lateral Sclerosis, 4
Ayurveda, 55-57, 61-62, 66-67, 115, 141
    as science, 57
    doshas (body types), 62, 66
    ideal day, 66-67

Bach Flower Remedies, 131, 133
Bedson, Scott, 37
Beyondananda, Swami, 16, 29, 43, 77, 126
Bicycles, 14, 49, 51, 117, 134
Bioacoustics, 121, 124, 131, 133
Bischofberger, Iren, 137
Body Memory, 58, 60
Brancale, Anthony, 119
Bruyere, Rosalyn, 142
Buxman, Karen, 32

Cameron, Julia, 44
Cane, 56, 68-72, 82, 103, 109-111, 125, 132, 134
Carter, Ellen, 28
Chakras, 60, 89
Chan, Dr. Jane, 9
Chelation, 100-101, 104-105, 110, 113-114, 124
    intravenous, 101, 106, 114
    oral, 107-108, 124
Cline, Manny, 78, 128
Comic Relief Telethon, 6
Comic Relief humor group, 6
Cousins, Norman, 142

Dentistry, ix, 94-95, 100, 102, 141
    Ammeter reading, 107
    Circaseptuan cycle, 102
    root canal tooth, 107-108
Dhonden, Dr. Yeshe, 51-53, 58, 78, 123
Diet, 47-49, 53, 63, 65, 67, 97, 113-117, 131, 133, 141
DMPS, 101-102
Dreams, 35, 47, 50, 114

Energy, i, xi, 10, 17-18, 21, 27, 30-31, 33, 43-44, 50-51, 53-54, 56, 58, 60, 63, 66, 69, 73, 75-77, 79-80, 84-92, 97, 100, 104, 106, 109, 111-112, 114, 116, 119-120, 123-125, 128-133, 137-138, 141-142
    human cell, 85
    long distance transmission of, 128-130
Exercise, 6, 17, 21, 29, 32, 69, 73, 77, 85, 90, 96, 111-112, 115, 119-120, 127, 131, 134, 137
    Qi gong, 33, 111-113, 122-125, 131, 133
    T'ai Chi, 53-55, 65, 85-86, 92, 97, 111, 115

walking, 1, 6, 37, 56, 61, 70-71, 81, 94, 104, 123, 130
Waterobics, 97
Yoga, ix, 25, 32, 55, 62, 66-67, 73, 77, 111, 127, 133, 142

Father issues, 59-61, 78-84
Fu, Dr. Ping, 122

Gawain, Shakti, 50
Gerson, Dr.Scott, 57, 73, 120
Gibran poetry, 11, 13
Ginseing, Korean, 125
Guan, Jamie, 53

Harris, John, 66, 114
Healing, 9-10, 24, 41, 46-50, 55, 57-60, 66-67, 73, 75, 77-78, 81, 84, 87-93, 105-106, 109-112, 116, 119-121, 127-128, 130, 132, 141-142
    prayer, 44, 51-52, 60, 109-110, 129
    subway, 1, 6-7, 18, 27, 43, 68-69, 71, 81, 103, 107-110
Healing Touch Inc., 58, 60, 87-92, 109, 112, 116, 120
Healing Works, 132
Herbs, 46-47, 49, 51-53, 58, 65, 74-75, 97, 113, 122-125, 128-130
    Angelica's, 117, 128
Homeless U.S. Veterans Association, 6, 28, 136
Huggins Diagnostic Center, 99, 101, 106, 115
Huggins, Dr. Hal, 94, 98
Humor, 1, 6, 11, 15-18, 20-22, 24-30, 33-34, 36, 39-41, 43, 46, 65, 67, 76, 80, 93, 97, 104-105, 108, 112-114, 116, 118, 121, 124, 126, 131-138, 142, 147
    and joy, 138
    and love, 6, 16, 136
    effect on body, 17, 24

    and communication, 17
    effect on mind, 20, 24-25, 29, 132
    intervention to nurse, 16-19, 26-27
    intervention to patient, 20-26, 31, 135-138
    self-applied, 90
    therapy, xi, 5-6, 9, 11, 16, 21, 28-31, 33-34, 37, 39, 53, 60, 69, 74, 76-77, 83-84, 100, 102, 112, 114, 120-121, 132, 134, 136-137, 142
    use in hospitals, 19-26

Improvisation, 29-30, 33-34, 137
    Gotham City Improv, 29

Johnson, Alexandra, 87
Jokes, 17, 20-21, 26, 32, 39, 137
    Recipe for telling, 39
Julian of Norwich, 46

Kataria, Dr. Madan, 32
Kipling poem, 35

Laminaria (sea vegetable), 129
Laughter Club International, 32
Levin, Dr. Warren, 100
Lymphatic drainage, 90, 120, 124

Massachusetts Eye and Ear Infirmary, 16
Massage, 63, 65, 73-75, 115-117, 119-120
Mentgen, Janet, 87, 120
Mercury, ix, 94-96, 98, 101-104, 110, 127, 130, 139
    exposure to, ix, 98
    toxicity, 94, 102, 108, 128

Metals, heavy, ix, 42, 48, 94-96, 100
    removal from teeth, 95-96, 98-104
    removal from body, 100-104
    sources of, 73, 103
    testing for, 100
Miller, Dr. Jean, 116
Music, 74, 116, 120-121

Natural Allergy Elimination Technique (NAET), 115-117, 124, 129
Neurological testing, 3-4, 15, 37, 57, 95, 96, 122-123
Norment, Doug, 60
Null, Gary, 98
Nursing, 3, 9, 16-17, 26, 41, 46, 83, 142
    and holistic practices, 58, 60, 86-92
    and need for humor, 17
    and spirit, 26, 57, 73
    frustrations of, 86
Nutritional supplements, 65, 113, 124

Panchakarma, xi, 67, 73-77, 87-88, 113, 119, 124, 131, 133
Primary Lateral Sclerosis, 43, 52, 61, 96, 101
    symptoms of, 57

Qi gong, 33, 111-113, 122-125, 131, 133

Richterman, Burt, 6, 27
Riluzol, 9, 43
Rumi poetry, 11, 14, 151

Singer, Susan, 47
Smiling, 8-9, 23, 40-41, 99, 110, 137

Spirit, 6-7, 11, 26-27, 31, 49-51, 57, 73, 78, 83, 87, 108-109, 115, 137
St. Vincent's Hospital, 37

Tache, Judith, 60
Tessier, Maria, 49
T'ai chi, 53-55, 65, 85-86, 92, 97, 111, 115
Transformational Breath work, 60
Tricycle, 82, 133-134

Valentina, 128-129
Veterans Administration Treatment Center, 28-34
Visualization, 25, 49-50, 65
    coming into reality, 134

WBAI Radio Station, 65, 98, 108, 111, 114, 120
Wedding, xi, 3, 8, 11
Wilson, Steve, 32, 33
Work, 1, 10, 15-16, 20, 23, 29-30, 33, 36, 42-43, 45-47, 50-51, 59, 61, 67, 78-81, 83-84, 87, 90-92, 95, 97, 104-105, 108, 114, 124-128, 130, 132, 136-137
    in bakery, 45-46
Workaholism, 81
Wylie, Elizabeth, 127

Author's Biography

▼

Florence Ditlow, is a registered nurse. Her patients repeatedly proved to her that surviving illness depends upon your attitude and your sense of humor. When she faced a mysterious illness, Florence used her sense of humor, in order to creatively achieve wellness.

She lives with Genady Filkovsky, her spouse, in Edgewater, New Jersey. You may contact Florence by e-mail: longinthetooth@att.net

0-595-24771-7